DOCTORS ENDORSE "EAT FOR HEALTH"

"Medicine is in great need of a paradigm shift in its approach to healthcare delivery. *Eat for Health* is an extraordinary book and can be an important catalyst for such a paradigm shift. It should be a must read for healthcare professional students, healthcare professionals, healthcare policy makers, and any individual seeking optimal health."

> — **Baxter Montgomery, MD, FACC**
> *Clinical Assistant Professor of Medicine*
> *University of Texas Healthscience Center,*
> *Houston, TX*

"A terrific, "non-diet" diet. Dr. Fuhrman explains precisely what you should eat and he makes it delicious. *Eat for Health* is effective, practical and sensible."

> — **Richard N. Podell, M.D., M.P.H.,**
> *Medical Director and Clinical Professor*
> *Department of Family Medicine*
> *UMDNJ-Robert Wood Johnson Medical School*

"As a physician, I follow Dr. Fuhrman's excellent recommendations myself and I have prescribed them to my patients with some wonderful results. *Eat for Health* is a great book for anyone who wants to see less of the doctor!"

> — **Anna Quisel MD**
> *Family Physician*
> *Wilmington, Delaware*

"Dr. Fuhrman's book summarizes a practical and effective method to live a long and healthy life – devoid of chronic disease and full of the vitality intended for us all by Mother Nature. Here is a chance to make your most important investment... the rest of your life!"

— **Matt Lederman, M.D.**
Board Certified Internal Medicine
Director of Transition to Health's Nutrition
and Wellness Program
Los Angeles, California

"Dr. Fuhrman's nutritional prescription is a greatly-needed antidote to the US way of eating which has become a leading cause of disease and premature death. Despite all the sophisticated medical technology available today, the sobering truth is that the greatest tools for preventing and reversing disease are your fork and spoon. This way of eating will greatly benefit those in poor health as well as healthy persons desiring optimal wellness and vitality. Further, unlike most weight-loss approaches based on "will-power" and difficult to sustain, Dr. Fuhrman's approach corrects the underlying causes of excessive hunger and cravings, resulting in permanent, naturally-occurring weight loss. I have had the privilege of personally seeing the tremendous disease reversal that occurs with this way of eating, and whole-heartedly recommend this book."

—**Tonja R. Nansel, PhD**
Investigator, Prevention Research Branch
Department of Epidemiology, Statistics,
and Prevention Research
National Institute of Child Health
and Human Development

"Dr. Fuhrman's message is scientifically valid, clinically proven, and very much worth considering for anyone who wants to really enjoy personal health. This prescription for health is both profound and broad in its effect."

—**T. Colin Campbell, PhD**
Professor Emeritus of Nutritional Biochemistry
Cornell University
Co-author, "The China Study"

NOW FLIP THIS BOOK OVER
TO GO BACK TO

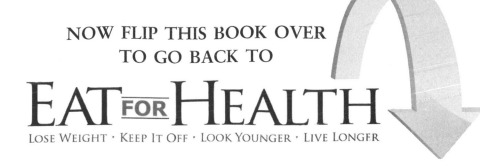

EAT FOR HEALTH

LOSE WEIGHT · KEEP IT OFF · LOOK YOUNGER · LIVE LONGER

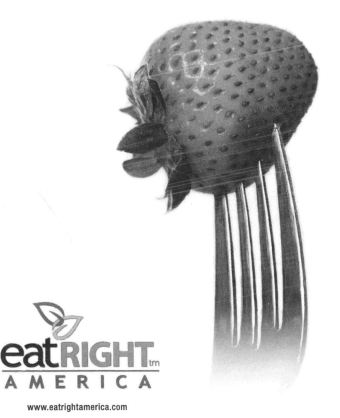

BOOK ONE
the mind makeover

eatRIGHTtm
A M E R I C A

www.eatrightamerica.com

"Dr. Fuhrman has done a magnificent job of synthesizing the essence of thousands of peer reviewed medical journal articles and devising a dietary program that can work miracles for your health! This man is a pioneer in preventive medicine."

—David W. Bullock, D.O.
Physical Medicine &Rehabilitation Specialist
Lawrence, KS, & Social Security Medical Consultant

"I love this book. It's hard to believe that Dr. Fuhrman could surpass his earlier book, *Eat To Live*, but he did. *Eat for Health* empowers us to make change. It is the only prescription that will ensure that our golden years remain golden and not riddled with disability and disease. Dr, Fuhrman's advice can enable you to achieve the same weight loss seen with gastric bypass surgery WITHOUT the surgery. A must read to "exercise" your taste buds and rev up your metabolic machinery."

—Deanna Cherrone, M.D.
Board Certified in Internal Medicine
Founder of Natural Health & Healing, LLC
Avon, CT

"Dr. Fuhrman's nutritional approach to the prevention and management of chronic disease is the most significant medical advance I have seen in my career as a physician."

—John V. Forrest, M.D.
Professor of Radiology, UCSD Medical School

"In *Eat for Health* Dr. Fuhrman has taken the most accurate information about nutrition today and made it understandable for anyone who is interested in being responsible for their own health. Dr. Fuhrman's food rating system— Aggregate Nutrient Density Index makes it easy to decide what to eat. Take this knowledge that's presented so clearly and live a healthy life."

—Deborah Pate, D.C., D.A.C.B.R.
Chiropractor and chiropractic radiologist
San Diego, CA

"If you took a pill every day that made you slimmer, healthier and reversed most disease processes in your body, you would call it a medical miracle. I have witnessed that Dr.Fuhrman's *Eat for Health* program can provide that miracle makeover that you have been looking for. Plus, it is a delicious and pleasurable way to eat. *Eat for Health* and create your own miracle—today"

—**Michael Klaper, M.D.**
Family and Emergency Room Physician
Author and Nutritional Researcher

"Follow Dr. Fuhrman's easy-to-understand formula in this book and start having the healthiest time of your life. Fad dieting has no long-term weight and health benefits, but when you eat high nutrient foods the results stick."

—**Gerald Deutsch, President**
National Health Association

"At last, a way to eat that can prevent and even reverse disease! And you will stay slim without dieting. Dr. Fuhrman shows us exactly what we need to do and why we need to do it. My wife and I do it! You are what you eat and if YOU don't take care of yourself...no one else can or will. Dr. Fuhrman teaches us nutritional excellence that can even prevent macular degeneration. Start now to live healthier and longer."

—**Stephen Lichtenstein, M.D.**
Attending Surgeon, Wills Eye Institute
Philadelphia, Pennsylvania

"Awesome! *Eat for Health* is the best, real-world tool I have seen yet for helping people pursue optimal health and/or deal with the majority of today's diseases. This approach is what "primary care" should be in modern healthcare. The "nutrient density" approach in *Eat for Health* is the cure for most of our diseases and our salvation from the fad diets that plague us. *Eat for Health* is both based on good science and very practical for real people, it could solve the healthcare crisis in America."

—**Marc Braman, MD, MPH**
Director of Lifestyle Medicine
Wellspring Medical Center

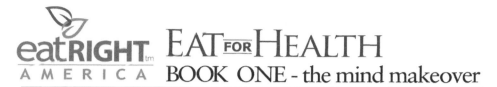

eatRIGHT™ AMERICA   EAT FOR HEALTH
BOOK ONE - the mind makeover

This scientifically proven system will enable you to lose your cravings and food addictions, while guiding your taste buds to prefer healthful foods over low-nutrient ones. Medical research proves this is the most effective weight loss method ever studied. Participants lost an average of 53 pounds—and kept it off!

Use high-nutrient foods to lose weight and keep it off, overcome disease, reverse diabetes, lower your blood pressure and cholesterol without medications, protect yourself against cancer and get more pleasure out of eating. *Eat For Health* will transform your thinking and empower you to improve your health. It can save your life.

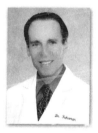

ABOUT THE AUTHOR

Joel Fuhrman, M.D., is a board-certified family physician specializing in lifestyle and nutritional medicine and a graduate of the University of Pennsylvania School of Medicine.

As one of the country's leading experts on nutrition and natural healing, Dr. Fuhrman has been featured in hundreds of magazines and on major radio and television shows, including: "Good Morning America," CNN, "Good Day NY," TV Food Network, and the Discovery Channel's "Second Opinion with Dr. Oz."

Dr. Fuhrman's recommendations are designed for people who want to achieve superior health, maintain effective weight control, and reverse and prevent disease. His most recent books include *Eat to Live, Cholesterol Protection for Life, Disease-Proof Your Child,* and Eat Right America's *Nutritarian Handbook.*

First Edition, Published March 2008

Copyright 2010 by Joel Fuhrman, MD

Contact:
Joel Fuhrman, MD
4 Walter Foran Boulevard, Suite 409
Flemington, NJ 08822

Printed in the United States
ISBN: 9780982554180

Publishers Note:
Keep in mind that results vary from person to person. Some people have a medical history and/or condition that may warrant individual recommendations and in some cases drugs and even surgery. Do not start, stop or change medication without professional medical advice, and do not change your diet if you are ill or on medication except under the supervision of a competent physician. Neither this, nor any other book, is intended to take the place of personalized medical care or treatment.

A small percentage of the names used have requested their names be changed.

Book Design: Robyn Rolfes — Creative Syndicate, Inc.

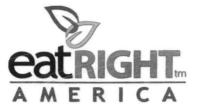

eatRIGHT™
A M E R I C A

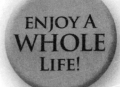

ENJOY A
WHOLE
LIFE!

You Can *Personalize* Your Nutritarian Plan with...

Eat Right America's Nutrition Prescription™

ERA's NUTRITION PRESCRIPTION IS THE NATION'S ONLY ONLINE, PERSONALIZED, EATING PLAN DESIGNED SPECIFICALLY TO ENSURE YOU GET THE NUTRITIONAL GUIDANCE YOU NEED TO ENJOY A WHOLE LIFE.

After a ten minute on-line survey the Nutrition Prescription will produce:

- A Personal Eating Assessment
- A Personal Disease Risk Evaluation
- A Personal Eating Plan
- A Personal Fitness Plan

- Customized Nutritional Recommendations that Meet Your Unique Needs
- 28 Days of Personal Emails to Support Your Plan
- 60 Days Free Access to the Eat Right America Community Website

The Nutrition Prescription is now available from the privacy of your own home.

TRY IT NOW!

A TWO-YEAR STUDY
OF THE HIGH NUTRIENT DIET
PRODUCED AN AVERAGE WEIGHT LOSS
OF 53 POUNDS.

For information on how to get started, visit:
www.EatRightAmerica.com/EatForHealth
or call
1-877-525-8384

BOOK ONE
the mind makeover

1

EAT FOR HEALTH

LOSE WEIGHT · KEEP IT OFF · LOOK YOUNGER · LIVE LONGER

Joel Fuhrman, M.D.

PUBLISHED BY
NUTRITIONAL EXCELLENCE, LLC.

This book is dedicated to all Americans suffering with chronic disease, who were told their problem was simply genetic and that drugs and interventions such as angioplasty and bypass surgery are the only answer.

Even though it is well accepted in the scientific literature that nutritional excellence has powerful therapeutic application, this information has not filtered down to the average American.

People need to know they have a choice. They have a right to know they do not have to suffer and die prematurely of medical conditions that are easily prevented and reversed via nutritional excellence.

So if you have high blood pressure, high cholesterol, diabetes, heart disease, peripheral vascular disease, reflux esophagitis, chronic headaches, irritable bowel syndrome, autoimmune disorders or other chronic medical conditions and you desire improved health, vitality and to free yourself of medical dependency this book is especially dedicated to you with the hope it will transform your health.

ACKNOWLEDGEMENTS

I had assistance from many people in developing this manual and especially with the recipes. My wife, Lisa reads everything I write and helps me immensely with great suggestions. The editor, Meghan Conaton did a great job of organizing the content for easy digestibility and Robyn Rolfes designed the cover layout, and look and feel. Robert Phillips researched and contributed to the development of the concepts relating social relationships and dietary change. My friend and co-founder of Eat Right America, Kevin Leville jointly developed the MANDI food scoring system with me, as well as other practical applications of this system that have patents pending. Linda Popescu, R.D. performed the nutritional analysis and painstaking scoring of every recipe, Janice McDonnell-Marra, my business manager, coordinated the team's efforts and assisted with every step.

I believe the recipes here are unique in that they make the healthiest foods in the world taste great. You have to see them and taste them to believe it! Many of the recipes are my family's favorites that my wife, Lisa and I have collected over the years. Others have been contributed by chefs working day in and day out tweaking and tasting every one multiple times. Robin Jeep, Allisa Shankoff, and Marian Fanok contributed to and tested every recipe in our office kitchen.

TABLE OF CONTENTS

FOREWARD
BY JOHN ABRAMSON, M.D.

Almost daily we hear news of exciting medical breakthroughs. We're barraged by drug ads trying to convince us we need medications to cure diseases we didn't even know we had. And our doctors' enthusiasm about prescribing the latest medicines, tests, and procedures is highly contagious. It's almost impossible not to get swept up in the expectation that we can count on the latest in medicine to protect and restore our health.

There is no doubt that modern medicine can be a God-send, and many of us have benefited from good medical care. But all this good news sounds too good to be true. And it is. The real story is that most of these "miracles" are being foisted upon the public, not because of the health benefits they bring to us, but because of the financial benefits they bring to the medical industries that manufacture these beliefs.

There is, however, a genuine scientific breakthrough that is readily available to you and it isn't expensive. It is the health-giving, disease-preventing power of a truly healthful eating-style. The one thing it does require, however, is that you reclaim responsibility for keeping yourself healthy.

According to both the prestigious Institute of Medicine and researchers from the Robert Wood Johnson Foundation, two-thirds of our health is determined not by the medical care we receive, but by our health habits and the environment in which we live. The problem is that there's a mismatch between what is being done to help us preserve our health and what the scientific evidence shows us would be a lot more effective. Nineteen out of 20 of our healthcare dollars are spent on biomedical interventions like medications, procedures, blood tests, x-rays and MRIs. These biomedical interventions use up all the time and resources that could also help us address the kinds of things that would dramatically improve our chances of staying healthy.

One example: Women can't avoid being confronted with the message that heart disease is their #1 killer and in order to protect themselves, they should "know their numbers." Of course we all know that this means knowing your cholesterol numbers, and we also know that this will lead many otherwise healthy women to be put on a cholesterol-lowering drug by their doctors. There are several things wrong with this common medical narrative:

1. Despite the National Cholesterol Education Program's guidelines for treating healthy women with cholesterol-lowering drugs when their risk hits certain thresholds, there has never been a single, randomized controlled, clinical trial (gold standard) that shows that women who don't already have heart disease or diabetes, benefit from taking a statin. (I know this sounds crazy, but I am the author of an article published in the British medical journal, The Lancet, in January of 2007 titled "Are Lipid-Lowering Guidelines Evidence Based?" that made exactly these points.)

2. Eating a healthy diet is three times more effective than taking a cholesterol-lowering statin drug for preventing a recurrent heart attack. Contrary to what is generally thought, the healthy diet doesn't help by lowering cholesterol that much. A healthful diet-style reduces the risk of heart disease by an assortment of other known and unknown mechanisms. Like a good magician, cholesterol-lowering marketing campaigns have focused our attention on cholesterol levels when we should be focused on the real goal: reducing the risk of heart disease and improving overall health.

3. One study followed 7300 healthy women for 31 years to see what risk factors contribute most to premature death. The contribution of elevated cholesterol to increased mortality rate was exactly zero. On the other hand, the Nurses' Health Study shows that women who follow five healthy habits develop 83% less heart disease and 91% less diabetes than women who

don't follow the healthy habits—eat a healthy diet, exercise regularly, don't smoke, don't drink heavily, and maintain a good body weight.

Surprisingly, only 3 out of 100 American women adhere to these healthy habits. We are investing most of our health care resources in lowering cholesterol with drugs instead of helping women adopt healthy lifestyles, which would be far more effective and less costly. Americans now spend about twice as much per person on healthcare as the other 21 wealthiest industrialized countries. Of course, there's little that's more important than health, so if this is what it takes to get the best healthcare in the world, then most people think the high cost of healthcare is a necessary evil. But it's not just the cost of American healthcare that's out of line. The really bad news is that for all the extra money we are spending, Americans not only don't have the best health, we have the worst among the citizens of the wealthiest 22 countries. According to the World Health Organization, Americans live an average of two and a half fewer years in good health than the citizens of these other countries.

Adding insult to injury, according to the World Health Organization, the efficiency of the American healthcare system (meaning how much health we get for the money we spend) ranks 72nd in the world! Can you imagine how long your employer would continue to buy services from a supplier that ranked 72nd in efficiency, was charging your company twice as much as your international competitors, and achieving inferior results?

Researchers from Dartmouth Medical School calculate that about one third of American healthcare expenditures are now devoted to services that don't improve health and may actually make things worse. This means that Americans are wasting more than $700 billion per year on unnecessary or harmful healthcare. To put this in perspective, the amount we are wasting each year on unnecessary or harmful medical care is more than the entire budget of the United States Department of Defense.

Corporations are struggling to purchase healthcare coverage for their employees and, by necessity, shifting costs to their workers in the form of higher monthly payroll deductions, higher deductibles and co-pays, and less coverage. As a result, the number of uninsured Americans is increasing by about one million every year and the majority of the recently uninsured are middle class, full-time workers. They and their employers can't afford health insurance.

We need to get to the bottom of the dysfunction in our national approach to health. The politicians don't want to address the real issues because most of them are dependent on contributions and other support from the healthcare industry. Most of the "experts" don't want to get to the real issues either, because they too have financial ties to the medical industry; same with universities, with medical journals, and even the media.

The "core lesion" (as we doctors say) is that medical knowledge itself is now produced and disseminated primarily for its profit-generating potential. I am not talking about the ads on TV or about the so-called non-profit groups that take large amounts of money from the medical industry. I'm not even talking about the free lunches that the drug companies' sales reps bring to doctors' offices to get them to listen to their sales pitches. Or about the continuing education lectures and seminars that doctors attend to maintain their licenses, which are overwhelmingly sponsored by the drug and other medical industries. This is where it gets really scary: I am talking about the clinical trials that are published in our most trusted medical journals. The majority of these studies are industry sponsored, and research shows that the odds are five times greater that these commercially sponsored clinical studies will conclude that the sponsors' drugs are the treatment of choice compared to non-commercially sponsored studies of exactly the same drugs!

To make matters worse, almost all of the articles in medical journals that influence the way that doctors practice medicine have commercial sponsorship. Between 1999 and 2004, for example, all but one of the 32 most influential articles that were published had commercial sponsorship. The commercial corruption of the sources of medical knowledge has become so overwhelming that the current editor of the Lancet and the recent editor of the British Medical Journal told the New York Times that "[Medical] journals have devolved into information-laundering operations for the pharmaceutical industry."

When the drug and other medical industries invest in research, their primary responsibility is not to optimize your health, but to maximize their shareholders' return on investment. In a medical system with proper oversight, these two goals would be the same—the profits made by private industry would be a direct reflection of their contribution to our health. But the oversight of the FDA, medical journals, universities, and academic physicians has all been seriously eroded by growing dependence on drug and other medical industry funding.

The end result is that the "knowledge" that your doctor receives from the sources that he or she has been trained to trust is distorted in two ways. First, the evidence is overwhelming that the conclusions presented in even the most trusted medical journals are biased in favor of their commercial sponsors. And second, in the same way that plants grow toward sunlight, the "knowledge" produced by commercially sponsored medical research grows towards the medical interventions that have the greatest potential to generate profits instead of the greatest potential to improve our health.

This may sound like dismal news, but understanding the truth points the way to enormous opportunities for you to take back control of your health (and for your employer to become a more intelligent purchaser of healthcare services). Your health is mostly in your control, but a guide is needed to show the way and protect you from getting distracted by all the commercial hype that surrounds health and healthcare.

For a healthier workforce and a healthier nation, both medically and economically, the information in this book is the solution. The solution to our health-care problem is not going to come from making better drugs or from better distribution of economic resources. It has to come from each of us taking better care of our health, so we avoid the need for medical interventions. For those of you taking medications, without addressing the dietary cause of your problem—this book is for you. For those of you who just want to live healthier and longer without medical disability and needless medical tragedies—this book is for you too. And for those of you who are concerned about the economic health of our nation—this book is for you as well.

This is why Dr. Fuhrman's work is so important. It is what we need to hear, well-researched, up-to-date, scientific information about healthy nutrition taught with wisdom and compassion. Not a fad diet, and not requiring great feats of self-denial, *Eat for Health* shows you how to take control of your dietary habits without going hungry and without denying yourself all of your favorite foods. The most fascinating aspect of this plan is that eating healthier can lead to greater, not less eating pleasure. You will quickly realize that you don't have to be a slave to unhealthy habits and you don't have to be controlled by the intense marketing for highly processed, calorie-dense, nutrient-poor foods.

Please accept my congratulations for reading this and deciding to take control of your health future. Study it well. Soon you will be enjoying a diet that will improve your health tremendously. You will have more energy and will be taking pride in the way that your body is responding to being fed well. *Eat for Health* has a powerful message, it may save your life.

John Abramson MD
Author, *Overdosed America:*
The Broken Promise of American Medicine
Clinical Instructor, Harvard Medical School

Prepare For A New You!

Congratulations on starting this program! Your decision to pursue superior health is one of the most important journeys you will ever undertake.

I developed *Eat for Health* after a comprehensive review of over 20,000 scientific studies on human nutrition over the last 20 years. I can say with certainty that this is the place to begin your nutritional turnaround. I have seen the effects of this plan in action on thousands of patients with a wide range of diseases and health concerns, from migraines and allergies to heart disease and diabetes, and the bottom line is, it works. The results over the years have demonstrated that this diet's foundation, nutritional excellence, is our most powerful intervention, not only to prevent disease, but also to reverse it and enable people to recover completely from most chronic degenerative illnesses. It is the path to medical wellness in your own life.

Nothing shows the power of this way of eating more than hearing from people who apply this knowledge and live it every day in their own lives. Throughout this book, beginning with Chapter One's selection of Medical Case Studies, you will find testimonies from a sampling of people from around the country who have changed their lives following this plan. They are from different backgrounds, are different ages, and had different reasons for beginning this journey, but they all now share excellent health. As you make your way through this book, take a moment to think about their stories and to discover the advantages that are possible when you eat right and make a commitment to your own health.

The physical change that you can create is one that your body was made to live. The body is a self-healing machine when you supply it with an optimal nutritional environment, and the information presented here is the fastest and most effective way to create that environment. If you have high blood pressure, high cholesterol, diabetes, heart disease, indigestion, headaches, asthma, fatigue, body aches, or pain—or you want to prevent yourself from developing these and other chronic conditions—this plan is for you. *Eat for Health* can enable you to avoid angioplasty, bypass surgery, and other invasive procedures. If you are not yet ill, it can make sure you never have a heart attack, stroke, or dementia in your later years. It can reduce and eventually eliminate your need for prescription drugs. In short, it can enable you to optimize your health and potentially save your life. And it can do all of this while increasing the pleasure you get from food.

Many of you have invested in this program to lose weight. I want to assure you that you will lose all the weight that you want, even if diets have failed you in the past. This is the most effective weight loss plan ever documented in medical literature and the results are permanent, not temporary. According to a recent medical study, the nutritional program presented in this book is the most effective way to lose weight, especially if you have a lot of weight to lose. The subjects, followed for two years, lost more weight than the subjects of any other study in medical history, and they kept it off.[1] More and more, new medical studies are investigating and demonstrating that diets rich in high-nutrient plant foods have a suppressive effect on appetite and are most effective for long-term weight control.[2] The healthiest way to eat is also the most successful way to obtain a favorable weight, if you consider long term results.

Many of my patients have lost up to 20 pounds in six weeks and that was just the beginning. However, this is nothing like your typical diet book because when the focus is on weight loss alone, the results are rarely permanent. Here, there is no calorie counting, portion-size measuring, or weighing involved. You will eat as much food as you want, however, and over time you will become satisfied with fewer calories. This is an eating-style that you will learn to enjoy forever. The goal here is to have the information change you in a natural fashion, so this becomes your preferred way of eating. To accomplish this, you will be presented with scientific, logical information that explains the connection between food and your health. By incorporating this information into your life and using the included meal plans and great-tasting recipes, you will shed pounds naturally and almost miraculously, merely as the side effect of eating so healthfully.

The reason the program works so well is because its success is hinged on knowledge. It takes time and effort to learn this body of knowledge, but that's because this program is not simply a quick fix. Once you have learned and practiced all of the information available to you, you will be a nutritional expert and the keys to successfull weight management will be in your hands—and your mind.

While weight loss is important, it is not our main goal. It is a pleasant and normal by-product on the road to the primary goal: great health. Superior health is marked by an exceptionally long and relatively disease-free lifespan, and countless studies reveal that people with superior health are slim. By teaching you how to achieve superior health, your ideal weight will follow naturally. You will understand the physical cravings that cause overeating, as well as the psychological factors that can help you change this pattern of consumption. Applying the information in this book to your life will help you achieve long-term success because it will create new, healthy behaviors that will eventually become effortless. It is so highly effective that it enables you to take control of your own health destiny.

What Is *Eat to Live*?

Eat To Live is the title of my bestselling book published in 2003. People all over the globe soon used that phrase to describe the overwhelmingly successful eating-style I created. I received a continuous barrage of e-mails and letters of gratitude describing miraculous changes in health thanks to the book. Those testimonies—some of which you will read in these pages—encouraged me to develop *Eat for Health*.

Developing *Eat To Live* and seeing the changes it caused in all of those people reinforced my knowledge that high-nutrient diets can restore the body to good health. Thousands of people lost dramatic amounts of weight without difficulty and never regained it back. More importantly, they recovered from diseases such as allergies, asthma, acne, headaches, high blood pressure, diabetes, reflux esophagitis, lupus, kidney insufficiency, angina, cardiomy-opathy, multiple sclerosis, and many more. The results and success stories are astounding.

I have long studied and utilized high-nutrient eating as a medical therapy, but even I have been surprised by the power of eating this way. For example, someone asked me on my website if my diet could make your hair turn brown after it had turned grey. I said, "Of course not," but then two people commented that it had happened to them. I could not believe it. Similarly, one of my patients had Hepatitis C before starting my eating-style. I didn't think this high-nutrient eating style would cure his hepatitis infection. However, after some time his Hepatitis C was completely gone. I had to repeat the blood tests three times to believe it. Those cases confirmed for me that eating this way could create medical transformations for millions of Americans.

My intention in writing this book was to make the principles of *Eat To Live* easier to incorporate in your life and to share the new lessons I've learned about the obstacles people have to making dietary changes. In addition, this book makes the *Eat To Live* principles more accessible to a larger audience. You will see that all people—sick or healthy, overweight or slim, young or old—can benefit from this plan because it creates the environment necessary for our bodies to thrive and experience what amounts to a miracle in our modern world: a long, disease-free life without heart disease, strokes, dementia, or even cancer.

Even though the information presented here is an extension of the nutri-tional and lifestyle program I laid out in *Eat To Live*, you do not have to read *Eat To Live* to understand this program. In this book, you will encounter the words, "*Eat To Live*," and when you do, keep in mind that it simply refers to a way of eating, a combination of food and lifestyle factors that I also refer to as my 'eating-style'. Everything you need to achieve your health and weight-loss goals is in the pages before you. All you need to do is read them and incorporate the information into your daily life.

Nutrients: The Basis of the Program

The eating-style that you will find in these pages is based on a central idea: Most people do not consume enough micronutrients on a daily basis. Because their micronutrient needs aren't met, they can't control food cravings and overeating. This deficiency also makes them more susceptible to the critical diseases and serious medical conditions that plague the American population.

Micronutrients are vitamins, minerals, and phytochemicals: valuable, but calorie-free parts of certain foods. My nutritional advice attempts to radically reduce your consumption of low-nutrient foods and radically increase your intake of high-nutrient foods. While the program will never ask you to count calories, for good health and a long, disease-free life we must seek to consume more nutrients from fewer calories. Basically, we must eat foods with a high nutritional bang per caloric buck. We will further discuss the relationship between nutrients and calories and how to determine the nutrient-density of foods in Phase One of this book.

Nutrient-density is the critical concept I use in devising dietary and nutritional advice to my patients and to the public. Adequate consumption of vitamins, minerals, and phytochemicals is essential for a healthy immune system and to empower your body's detoxification and cellular repair mechanisms that protect you from cancer and other diseases.

Perhaps not surprisingly, most of the foods that have a high nutrient-density are straight from nature, primarily fruits and vegetables. Therefore, these foods play major roles in our journey to great health. Nutritional science in the last 20 years has demonstrated that colorful plant foods contain a huge assortment of protective compounds, most of which are still being studied by scientists. Many newly discovered and still unidentified compounds in nutrient-rich food work in fascinating ways to facilitate the removal of toxins from the body, detoxify carcinogens, repair DNA damage, and reduce free radical formation. Only by eating an assortment of natural foods that are nutrient-rich can we access the diversity of these elements that are necessary to protect ourselves from common diseases.

You Are the Cure

I have been part of the medical community as a family physician for almost 20 years, and I can tell you that drugs and doctors cannot grant you excellent health and protection from disease and suffering. Almost every doctor knows this. The most effective health-care is self-care. Reading this book, practicing the plan and mastering its techniques will deliver the best possible self-care to you: nutritional excellence. The nutritional excellence I'm describing can prevent and even reverse most medical problems within three to six months. This is a bold claim, but the facts, supported by scientific research and literature, show that most medical problems and medical tragedies we face in the modern world are the result of nutritional folly. Our American diet has resulted in a sickly nation with the majority of people taking prescription drugs by the time they reach the age of 50. Your body is made of the foods you have eaten, and when you eat the standard American diet (SAD), you get the diseases that most other Americans get.

Fifty percent of Americans die of heart attacks and strokes. You don't have to be one of them! Twenty-eight million Americans suffer from the crippling pain of osteoarthritis. You don't have to be one of them! Thirty-five million Americans suffer from chronic headaches. You don't have to be one of them! You simply do not have to be sick.

We consider it normal to lose youthful vigor in our thirties, carry 30 to 40 extra pounds, live with chronic illness in our late forties and fifties, only to live our last decades completely dependent on others. This should not be considered normal. This is the result of a life-long pattern of unhealthy living and misguided information. We should look forward to enjoying an active life into our nineties. This seems like an outrageous expectation because most people spend a lifetime consuming an unhealthy diet. They have yet to make the connection that we are what we eat and that ill health in the later years of our lives is the result of our earlier, poor choices.

I have cared for more than 10,000 patients, most of whom first came to my office unhappy, sick, and overweight, having tried every dietary craze without success. After following this educational program for superior health and weight loss, they shed the weight they always dreamed of losing and they kept it off. For the first time in their lives they had a diet plan that didn't require them to be hungry all the time. Most importantly, they were able to eventually discontinue their medications. When you learn and follow this program of eating it is possible to:

- Never have a heart attack or a stroke

- Avoid dementia in later life

- Dramatically reduce your chance of getting cancer

- Prevent and heal digestive problems such as reflux, dyspepsia, constipation, and hemorrhoids

- Prevent and often resolve erectile impotence, high blood pressure, and other circulatory impairments

- Prevent and reverse diabetes (type two) and high cholesterol, at first lessening the need for drugs and eventually resolving these conditions

- Age slower, live longer, and maintain youthful vigor, intelligence, and productivity into the later years

Some people may be skeptical that I can make such radical claims, but these statements are supported by medical science and thousands of clinical patient case histories. The reversal of dietary-caused diseases occurs in a relatively short time and is easily observed by anyone following my program. However, don't make any decisions about starting the program yet. You first have to know much more about this. When you are ready to commit yourself to achieving superior health, I promise to make it almost impossible for you to fail.

About These Books
Eat for Health is designed to make this eating-style easy and fun by combining my relentless research and hands-on experiences with motivational exercises and mouth-watering recipes. I have developed and used this information with thousands of patients over the years with remarkable results.

The book that you are currently holding, Book One, provides all of the information, knowledge, history, tips, and techniques that you will need to understand each of the four phases of the program, practice their tenets, incorporate them into your daily life, and continue using them for long-term success. In it, you will learn that you have control over your health and weight. You will be pleasantly surprised to learn that you are not at the mercy of your genes or the pharmaceutical companies. You will also learn more specifically about why certain foods are more dangerous to our bodies than others and how you can learn to increase your enjoyment of the foods that are the most nutritious.

The companion to this book, Book Two, is a workbook and cookbook, intended to help you practically implement the program. The second book is based on graduated phases that correspond to the four phases presented in Book One. Each phase incorporates more nutritional principles to disease-proof your body as you learn more about this eating-style. The fourth and last phase is the most effective eating-style for reversing disease and maximizing health and longevity. While Phase Four is optimal, any level will bring you closer to your health goals and if you are overweight, you will still see dramatic benefits with all phases.

Each of the four phases in this program is, in fact, a separate nutritional plan. With the help of my staff, including world-class chefs, I have designed weekly menu plans with recipes for each phase. You can remain in any phase as long as you like. As you learn more and work with these books, your taste buds will gradually realign themselves and actually become stronger and more discriminating. As you become healthier, you will lose your psychological dependence on unhealthy foods. One of the ways in which *Eat for Health* is unique and revolutionary is that it is based on the idea of a gradual implementation of an increasingly higher micronutrient content in a person's diet. Where many diets ask you to go cold turkey on certain foods, or make the first weeks of their plans the hardest, this program is designed so you can make smaller changes first. As you increase your knowledge and preference for healthy foods, you can choose to move forward—all at your own pace. After you learn more of the science, practice the dietary modifications, and make some of the recipes, you can see the benefits and then challenge yourself with the next phase.

While it may be tempting to immediately begin trying the recipes and using the meal plans in Book Two, I strongly urge you only to move forward in the phases of Book Two after reading at least the corresponding information in Book One. While you may only choose to follow Phase One or Phase Two of Book Two, all of the information presented in Book One will help you in your efforts. Trying to live by this eating-style without understanding the intricacies of how and why it works will likely leave you with one more failed attempt at dietary change. At best, the benefits won't be permanent.

The recipes included in Book Two incorporate the healthiest, most nutrient-dense foods in the world to greatly increase the life-sustaining properties of your diet. *Eat for Health* will teach you an eating-style, not a calorie-counting formula. Do not focus on calories or portion sizes. Instead focus on increasing your intake of disease-protective nutrients with healthy foods.

I want to repeat that for clarity. The focus here is on learning about the disease-protective compounds in natural foods and how you can deliciously eat more and more of these foods. As you eat more of them, you will lose your food cravings, and you will automatically eat less unhealthy and fattening foods. If you are overweight, your weight will fall dramatically.

In the process, you will be enjoying some of my favorite recipes that rival the offerings at quality restaurants. This is not about deprivation! Rather, it is about living and experiencing life to its fullest. As you increase your intake of nutrient-dense foods and replace unhealthful foods, you will, over a period of time, reset your internal taste preferences and hunger drive. Once this happens, you will be amazed at how easy it becomes to follow my plan and maintain your ideal weight forever, without dieting.

Using This Book

This book is broken down into four phases that correspond to the four dietary phases in Book Two, which contains a meal planner and a recipe and shopping guide. These four phases take you on a journey into eating a great tasting diet that is very different from the diet most Americans eat today. The four-phase approach with four different menu plans allows you to adjust to this eating-style gradually. As you learn more about high-nutrient foods in each phase, the corresponding meals in Book Two will become healthier by increasing the micronutrients you consume with disease-fighting foods.

Go at your own pace. Read Phase One of this book and then use the plans and recipes in Phase One of Book Two. But of course, continue on reading the subsequent chapters and phases in Book One while you are living with the phase one eating recommendations. When you think you're ready to move forward to the second level in Book Two, return to Book One and refresh your knowledge of the Phase Two chapters before moving on. Do the same for the other phases as you feel comfortable, or read through this book completely, and then determine which phase is right for you to start before jumping in.

Regardless of how you choose to use this book, I advise you to master the material and exercises in each phase before moving on to the next one. The goal of this program is to teach you to eat healthfully, enjoy it, and learn to prefer a healthy eating-style instead of a disease-promoting one. Don't decide now whether you think you can do it or whether you want to make all these changes. Learn the information before making a judgment; give the information a chance to work.

After you finish Phase One of this book you will see and understand why the menus are constructed the way they are. It may be that the change from the way you eat now to the first phase of this eating-style is a big one. If so, you can make this first big change and stop there, or you can continue to change even more as you go on with the rest of the book. It's all up to you.

Taking the initial step to transform your health and well-being is a big one. It takes initiative, and you must make a commitment if you want the astonishing results that are possible. The objective is for you to gradually prefer this type of eating as you learn more and more from the phases. I hope to be able to change your food preferences so that you will eventually prefer the healthiest foods. You may think that this will require a miracle, but what you will learn in this book will make it a reality.

Along the way, you will find a series of dietary exercises that will help you prefer healthy eating. Rather than working your muscles, they are exercises with food that will strengthen your digestive system, stretch your palate, and allow effortless weight loss without dieting. This is an innovative, new concept because this is not a diet; it is simply the healthiest way to eat and live.

Using Book Two
Book Two—the food guide, recipe guide and menu planner—contains four separate phases of healthy eating intended to practically and efficiently create your complete health makeover. Each phase of menus takes you to a new level of nutritional excellence. To help you see your progress, each of the foods in Book Two is scored. These numbers are a way to quantify the nutritional content of a variety of different foods. We will further discuss these numbers and how to use them in Phase One of Book One.

The purpose of this scoring system is not to have you count and calculate every food you eat. Rather, it is a teaching tool that enables you to compare and recognize a super-healthy diet from a moderately-healthy one. By seeing the scores in the recipes and menus, you can understand the difference between the four phases and you can see a tremendous difference between this program and any other diet plan or nutritional advice. It lets you see food in a different light, like putting on a special pair of glasses that enables you to immediately calculate the nutritional value of your diet. By studying the nutrient-density score of what you choose to put in your mouth, you can better recognize what a diet that is heart attack and cancer protective looks like. Do you want to lower your risk of heart disease by 30 or 40 percent? Or do you want to lower your disease risk by nearly 100 percent? It will be up to you to decide, but you will be amazed how few nutrients are earned from eating a dietary pattern similar to other Americans. This will help motivate you to increase the nutritional density of your diet, as you will then be able to visualize the characteristics of the eating-style that is richest in disease-fighting nutrients.

Remember, by the time you finish reading this book and studying the materials, you will be able to instantly distinguish high-nutrient foods from low-nutrient foods. You will know how to make a meal or pick foods in a restaurant of high nutrient density. However, the purpose of the scoring system is NOT to have you be fanatical about counting points and scoring foods. You do not have to carry around a calculator and a pad to monitor your nutrient scores. The intention is that you look at the way I calculate scores, understand it, and understand the way the recipes are constructed to increase their nutrient density. Then, you can do what I do, which is to naturally enjoy foods that score high on the nutrient density line and, in so doing, eat to increase your health.

This Is a Different Diet World

Get ready for an exciting three months of your life. If you follow this program for that time—whether through all four phases or only into Phase One or Two—you will experience a personal transformation that is only possible when you eat for health. You will be thrilled with how easily your weight drops and at the subtle changes you experience in your physical and emotional well-being. You will feel better than you have in years.

I know how frustrating it is to dive into a promising diet only to meet with failure. You blame yourself, which sets up a vicious cycle of guilt and punishment. This expresses itself through self-defeating behavior. Most people who have been through this cycle have given up on the idea of reaching their ideal weight. It seems impossible and their failure in the past reinforces this. That will not be the case here. Mediocre expectations yield mediocre results, so you must, right now, raise your expectations. Give this program a true test and follow it as directed, and I am confident you will get different results than you have in the past. You will not only lose your excess weight, but you will also see both subtle and dramatic improvements in your health. You will lower your cholesterol, triglycerides, and blood pressure. If you have adult-onset (type two) diabetes, it will improve and can eventually resolve. Most people are amazed as symptoms such as migraines, acid reflux, and indigestion disappear. You will experience the power of health.

I feel strongly that this is the healthiest diet for disease-protection and longevity, and, if you are significantly overweight, it is also the most safe and effective way to lose a dramatic amount of weight. It works for those who have failed at losing weight or achieving their dietary goals in the past. Studies have shown that only three out of 100 people who attempt to lose weight actually succeed. The problem is not people. The problem is that most weight-loss approaches focus on reducing calories. That winds up reducing nutrients simultaneously, which is predictive of eventual failure.

The cuisine designed for nutritional excellence is radically different from other plans because you eat a lot of food. Forget calorie counting and traditional diets. Don't panic because you feel full and satisfied; this is normal. If you are overweight, you will still lose weight. Your body appreciates the nutrients and will reward you with optimal health and an ideal weight.

> ## CAUTION:
> This program is so effective at dropping your weight, blood pressure, and blood sugar that medication adjustments will be necessary so that you are not over-medicated. If your blood sugar or blood pressure improves dramatically and medications are not reduced or eliminated, it could be harmful to your health. Please consult your physician.

Be One of the Few, Not the Many

Like the classic victim, we actually grow to love those things that are killing us—in this case, food. This phenomenon is known as addiction and an addiction to certain foods can be just as deadly as many other addictions. However, if you are reading this, it is not too late to change. I can show you how to get rid of the food addictions sabotaging your health.

Since you have purchased this program, you are probably interested in the relationship between what you eat and your health. It is likely you are already attempting to eat differently than those around you. The secret to achieving spectacular results is your willingness to exchange the fossilized, limiting beliefs held by most Americans for new and wonderful expectations. I offer you this simple idea: if you adopt this program, you will achieve your ideal weight, slow down the clock of aging, and prevent and even reverse disease, all at the same time. While doing this, you will also discover a level of enjoyment in eating that you have never imagined. It all begins with a state of mind, but you first must be open to the possibility that this can happen.

Your success is dependent on your willingness to learn. It is okay if you don't want to adopt everything in this program or even agree with everything you read at first. The way to get the most out of these books is to read both books completely. I recommend you suspend decision making at first. It is best if you wait until you have learned more, then you will be in an educated position to decide if you really do disagree with something and why. Try not to let what you have learned in the past cloud your learning here; nutritional science has changed dramatically in recent years. This scientific, nutritional program was designed after years of studying thousands of articles from the scientific literature, seeing the most effective nutritional interventions used by other physicians around the world, and observing and testing these methods with my patients. The preponderance of the evidence all points in the same direction: the program works and it works best for those who understand it best. Read, practice the exercises, and ask questions. Those that learn this program well typically find they achieve remarkable results.

Finding Your Motivation
You are what you eat. To be your best, you must eat the best. Perhaps you already know this, but it doesn't always make it easy to live that way. I will teach you new nutritional principles to enable you to think and grow healthy. I can also teach you to prefer to eat healthfully if you give me that chance, but motivation is key to starting the program and sticking with it.

On a scale of 1 to 10, rate the most compelling reasons you have for eating healthfully:

____I want to recover from a chronic illness, such as high blood pressure, diabetes, headaches, or high cholesterol.

____I want to protect myself from developing a dangerous disease.

____I want to prevent the deterioration in health, physical, and mental abilities that are typically considered a normal part of aging.

_____ I want to lose weight and look and feel better.

_____ I want to increase my energy and reduce fatigue.

_____ I want to improve the health of my family.

_____ I want to improve my physical fitness.

_____ I want protection from frequent bouts of infectious disease.

_____ I want to have better digestion.

_____ I want to have better sexual enjoyment and performance.

_____ I want to look and feel younger.

_____ I want to have a better emotional outlook on life.

_____ I want to live longer.

_____ I want to live without medical interference and hospitalizations.

_____ I want to avoid surgery or prescription medication.

_____ I want to reduce my dependency on medication.

_____ I want to save money on health care and prescription drugs.

Each time you feel some difficulty with the eating-style in this book, each time you want to revert back to your old ways of eating, each time you slip-up on the program, each time you believe this level of health is unattainable for you, come back and look at this page. Habits are hard to break and the way you eat is a habit. Remind yourself of how important these things are and why they are more than adequate motivation for continuing to learn, practice, and live with the goal of nutritional excellence.

Getting Started

Take your time ingesting the information presented in both of these books. Read them more than once and live with the information. If you have a copy of the audio version, listen to the CDs as well as reading the book. It is best to both listen and read, even if the material is redundant. The degree of redundancy here is purposeful and part of making certain information stick. The idea is for the information to become so familiar that you can recall it to a conscious level whenever you need to use it.

From Phase One to Phase Four, the dietary program changes in intensity. Getting through Phase Four does not mean you must live its eating-style perfectly every day, but if you put it into action it represents a degree of practice and mastery that has resulted in developing a set of skills that you will use for the rest of your life.

In going through this program, know that you are not alone. The cases that you will read throughout this book will remind you of that, but there are thousands of people from all over the globe who are utilizing these dietary principles. You will have the help of a community of like-minded people via **www.EatRightAmerica.com**, where you will communicate with thousands of others who are eating for health. My staff and I are committed to teaching, working, supporting, encouraging, listening, and answering you along the way. We are going to make sure you won't fail if you truly desire to succeed at this.

I urge you to take this program seriously, study it, and put it to work in your life. If you do, you will be rewarded with a healthy, almost disease-proof body, and you will naturally gravitate towards your ideal weight without counting calories, measuring portions, or eating only thimble-sized amounts of food.

Reaching your goals is no accident. Success requires thoughtful, directed action. We applaud the professional athlete whose precise moves are graceful and appear effortless. What we don't see are the years of physical training, the thousands of hours of practice, and the power of concentration that made it all possible. People who successfully reach their goals have worked diligently to reap the rewards. The same is true for attaining true health. So let's get started.

CHAPTER ONE

THOUSANDS OF SUCCESS STORIES

Eat For Health is the only eating style that will allow you to shed pounds while you reverse existing diseases and protect yourself from future health problems. In the following pages, you will learn about the science that makes this way of eating successful in fostering your health, and you will discover how to live this diet in your own life. However, what I often find even more convincing than the scientific data is seeing the results from patients who have followed my plan. For the past 16 years, I have been recommending the fundamentals of this diet to the patients in my medical practice, the readers of my previous book, and people who have reached out to me from around the world. In that time, I have seen the transformative power of practicing an eating-style focused on high-nutrient foods, the core of this plan. Hearing from people who have lived this plan and seen these changes in their own lives is thrilling.

Below is a small sampling of the thousands of emails and letters that I have received from my patients and from people who have followed my nutritional advice and discovered the transformative power of this way of eating. The illnesses and weight problems detailed below vary greatly, but all of these individuals found that the power of prescription medicine was nothing compared to the power of nutrition. Browse through their stories, hear them in their own words, and let their personal experiences inform and motivate you in your quest for great health. In seeing what this plan has done for their lives, you will see better what the *Eat for Health* plan can do for you, and you will be ready to implement it in your own life.

CARDIOVASCULAR ISSUES

"Five years ago, at the age of 49, my husband Don appeared to be in perfect health, but then he began to experience pressure in his chest. We found out that his left anterior descending artery was 95 percent blocked and his cholesterol was 259 with an LDL of 178. He had a stent placed, remained under the care of cardiologists, and was taking cholesterol lowering drugs, high blood pressure medications, and blood thinners. He tried to eat more carefully too, but he began having chest discomfort again and was found to have further heart disease.

This time, while waiting to have more invasive procedures performed, a friend of ours who is a doctor told us about the work Dr. Fuhrman was doing and encouraged us to see him as quickly as possible.

When we first met him, we were so impressed with the time Dr. Fuhrman spent with us, reviewing Don's history and sharing a wealth of information in a way that we could understand. We returned home with all the tools we needed to get us started on the journey to regaining health. We thoroughly enjoyed *Eat To Live* and immediately began to implement the program. We were amazed at the results.

Within two weeks Don had lost twelve pounds and his blood pressure dropped so low he no longer needed medications. Now he is 20 pounds lighter, his chest pains are resolved, and he was able to discontinue all his medications. His LDL cholesterol went from 163 while he was on medication to 103 off medication—and I lost 10 pounds as well! We both want to thank you for helping us understand how important it is to 'Eat To Live' by giving our bodies the food we need for proper nutrition. We just can't thank you enough for everything."

Laura and Don Klase
Orefield, Pennsylvania

LUPUS

"When I was 32 years old, I developed a rash on my face, and my body felt stiff and sore. The joint pain in my hands and shoulders continued to worsen, and my wrists felt like someone had hit them with a hammer. I saw a rheumatologist who prescribed an anti-inflammatory drug and blood work. It indicated that I had lupus. At first I thought, 'Good news. I have a diagnosis, so now I can do something about it.' I became discouraged when I was told there is no known cure for lupus. I would have to live with the disease and be on medication, including steroids, for the rest of my life. I was also told that I could experience serious organ damage, need a kidney transplant, and die. In addition, the medicine would make me gain weight and be puffy.

This information was not acceptable to me. I searched for answers, and, after trying other things with no success, I found Dr. Fuhrman. I traveled from Virginia to his office in New Jersey. I followed his advice regarding eating a high-nutrient diet, and, within a few months, I had made a complete recovery from lupus. For the first time in years, I looked and felt great.

I visited my old rheumatologist because I thought he would be impressed with my story. When I told him about my experience and my newfound health he wrote 'Spontaneous Recovery' on my chart and dismissed me rudely. So, when a doctor tells you that it has not been proven that diet has any effect on lupus, keep in mind that he may never have listened to people who told him otherwise. Today, lupus is not part of my life. I play tennis and compete on a local team, and no one would guess that I was ever in so much pain."

Robin Zelman
Charlottesville, Virginia

LUPUS WITH KIDNEY INVOLVEMENT

"In March 2004, my niece Julisa developed a rash. It was treated as poison ivy with topical medications. When the problem persisted, tests revealed kidney damage and stage-four lupus. She was placed on immunosuppressive drugs and steroids, creating very difficult side effects for a teenage girl. Desperate for alternative treatments, Julisa's mother and I searched for lupus information and found out about Dr. Fuhrman. He explained the benefits of natural, balanced nutrition and first prescribed a high-nutrient diet to improve Julisa's immune system. We were very skeptical, so we also took Julisa to a kidney specialist who told us that she was soon facing complete and inevitable kidney failure and would need dialysis. He placed Julisa on the national kidney transplant list.

We struggled with the options. On one hand, Julisa would endure a weekly routine of dialysis sessions and eventual kidney failure if a transplant wasn't found. On the other hand, she and the family would have to completely change our eating habits to comply with Dr. Fuhrman's program, and we weren't sure it was going to work. We finally decided to treat her lupus with Dr. Fuhrman's approach. Under his care she improved so quickly that he was able to gradually discontinue all of her medications. Amazingly, within a few months blood and urine testing revealed absolutely no trace of lupus in Julisa's system. Her kidney function has returned to normal. When we returned to the pediatric rheumatologist for a final check-up, he said he had never seen a case where the medications worked so well. He didn't even know we were able to slowly discontinue and then stop all the medications, and the results were all because of Dr. Fuhrman's nutritional program! It was a miracle."

Rosario and Julisa Taveras
Paterson, New Jersey

ASTHMA, MIGRAINES AND HIGH BLOOD PRESSURE

"By the age of 43, I was a physical mess. I was 70 pounds over-weight, asthma had become a constant nuisance in my life, and I had developed high blood pressure, acid reflux, and an irregular heartbeat. I was especially concerned because heart problems cost both my parents their lives at young ages. I was on blood pressure medications, four Tums, and two different inhalers. I also frequently required oral steroids. I was sent to a dietician who told me I would lose 10 pounds if I changed from drinking Coke to Diet Coke. For years I saw an allergist once a week for allergy shots. Then I started experience violent migraines on a frequent basis, which was the last straw. One day a friend gave me a news-paper article about Dr. Fuhrman's work and I called his office immediately.

Dr. Fuhrman's advice totally transformed my life and the lives of many of my friends. Six years later, I no longer have headaches. I have not needed asthma medications in years and I do not have high blood pressure anymore. I have lost 70 pounds and kept it off. I thank God for my good health and the high energy level I experience everyday. I realize that all my years of medical problems were self-caused by my food choices. Now my husband and I enjoy each meal from a repertoire of delicious, healthy recipes, and I can't imagine living any other way."

Linda Castagna
Milford, New Jersey

SARCOIDOSIS

"I was generally thin until I turned 32; then I gained 30 pounds almost overnight. At age 34, I began having labored breathing and was diagnosed with sarcoidosis. The disease caused significant scarring over a large area of my lungs. I began the standard treatment of a biopsy and steroids.

Another three years and 20 pounds later, my life changed when the button on my last comfortable pair of pants snapped and the zipper broke. It was funny and embarrassing, but deadly serious all at the same time. That day I decided I had to change and went to the bookstore to find some answers. I stumbled upon Dr. Fuhrman's book, and it made sense to me.

Six months later, I was 60 pounds lighter. Then my wife noticed a lump on my neck. It had been there for years, but without all my fat obscuring it, it was now readily visible. I had assumed that my gasping was the result of the sarcoidosis, but it turned out I had a massive thyroid cyst blocking my windpipe and cutting off my air supply. The doctors decided that it needed to come out.

Prior to surgery, I had an MRI and the doctors found I had no traces of sarcoidosis. It had completely cleared up, just as Dr. Fuhrman had predicted. The surgery was problematic and I went into anaphylactic shock because the walls of my thyroid were stretched to the limit. I almost died, but more sobering was the fact that if I hadn't followed Dr. Fuhrman's advice, the cyst would have remained obscured and burst on its own.

I am now 46 years old; I run 20 miles each week and have unbelievable stamina. My systolic blood pressure went from 140 to 108, and my current LDL cholesterol level is 40. I feel great, look 10 years younger than I did two years ago, and take no medications. You too can achieve your ideal weight, reverse disease, and delay the aging process!"

Bob Phillips
Morrestown, New Jersey

PSORIASIS AND PSORIATIC ARTHRITIS

"I was desperate when I traveled to New Jersey to see Dr. Fuhrman. I had been diagnosed with psoriatic arthritis and had suffered from open skin lesions and full body itchiness for years. I followed his advice to the letter. He put me on a special eating plan, and, after about three months, I started to get better. My legs and arms cleared up first. My body healed from the extremities inward, and six months later my psoriasis was totally gone. My doctors are amazed. Today my skin is completely clear with no itchiness or blotches, and I have no more arthritic pain. Recent blood tests show I no longer have the blood test markers that show inflammation. I cannot fully express what this recovery means to me. I am so grateful that Dr. Fuhrman insisted I could be helped and then guided me to wellness."

Jodi O'Neil
Cary, North Carolina

POLYMYALGIA AND FIBROMYALGIA

"I developed joint pains when I was 40 years old and then found out I had high blood pressure and high cholesterol. I went on the Atkins diet and my cholesterol shot up to over 300. My body aches and pains worsened and I was diagnosed with polymyalgia rheumatica and then fibromyalgia, a condition of chronic pain. I couldn't sleep well. I couldn't even sit on the toilet without severe pain. I took medications, steroids, and even used magnets, but nothing helped. I prayed and got to the point where I didn't even want to live if my life had to be like this.

Then a co-worker told me about the best health book she had ever read. It was *Eat to Live*. I read it in two days, and I still read it over and over again like a textbook. It has been two years since

I first got the book and today I am well. I can even work out at the gym four times a week. Many people think that eating unhealthy food is the most important thing, but I have learned that feeling great is even more important. I am 66 and I feel better than I did when I was 30."

Suzanne Demeo
South Orange, New Jersey

DIABETES AND DIABETIC RETINOPATHY

"Before I read Dr. Fuhrman's book I weighed 205 pounds and had diabetes for seven years. The information enabled me to lose 60 pounds and get rid of my diabetes, high blood pressure, and high cholesterol without medication. My LDL cholesterol went from 168 to 73 in five months, and I successfully dropped my weight to 143 pounds. The most amazing thing is that my ophthalmologist had told me that I required laser surgery to treat diabetic retinopathy, but after changing my diet he found that the damage was no longer there and I didn't require surgery. I am extremely grateful because I know Dr. Fuhrman has added many quality years to my life."

Martin Milford
Santa Rosa, California

SEVERE MIGRAINES AND FATIGUE

"Our daughter Renee has been plagued by headaches since she was five. They intensified when she was 11 and from that point on she suffered tremendously from the pain and the treatments she had to endure. In addition to an arsenal of drugs, she was hospitalized four times and even received intravenous drugs; nothing worked.

We went to chiropractors, nutritionists, dentists, acupuncturists, and rheumatologists, but nothing helped. Renee was not able to remain in school. She was tutored at home when she felt up to it, but most of the time she simply could not get out of bed.

As you can imagine, this had a profound impact on Renee and our family. She was forced to give up sports, trips, friends, school, and just being a kid. Twice she talked about not wanting to live anymore. As a result, she began seeing a counselor to help her deal with this life-altering illness.

I did not consider Renee an unhealthy eater, but at her first visit to Dr. Fuhrman he tested her level of antioxidants and carotenoids and found them to be extremely low. He explained that Renee's deficiencies of these nutrients were preventing her body from effectively removing metabolic wastes and other toxins. He told us it would take about three months for her to get well. We were highly skeptical, but Renee gave it her best shot. Our entire family ate Dr. Fuhrman's vegetable-based diet and truly enjoyed the recipes.

After one month I was still concerned because Renee did not seem better and was still suffering. I called Dr. Fuhrman and he reminded me that getting the nutrients into Renee's bloodstream did not mean those nutrients were concentrated in her skin, brain, and other tissues.

After three months, Renee was her old self again. She was smiling all the time and her headaches were almost totally gone. Her energy and personality returned, she has resumed school, and she's back doing sports again. I cried with joy when I saw Dr. Fuhrman again. He has given us our daughter back."

Janine Kranor
Oakland, New Jersey

ULCERS

"For approximately a year before consulting with Dr. Fuhrman, our daughter Caitlin suffered from progressive fatigue, severe acne, and chronic stomach upset. It caused numerous absences from school, which was troubling because Caitlin was an honor student who had always done well academically. After seeing several doctors with no diagnosis, Caitlin became exceedingly frustrated and asked us to enroll her in counseling for stress management. We began counseling as a family.

Caitlin's symptoms worsened and she was eventually diagnosed with ulcers. Six weeks later, we learned that the tests revealed an alarmingly high presence of the antibodies that fight bacterially-based ulcers. According to the doctor, Caitlin probably had the bacteria in her stomach for more than a year. He immediately prescribed a course of four antibiotics taken simultaneously, which destroyed her digestive system. She was worse than ever.

We asked our counselor to recommend a physician who practiced nutritional medicine and we were led to Dr. Fuhrman. He immediately put Caitlin on a cleansing diet with lots of green vegetables and high-nutrient soups, but no medication of any kind. Over those first two months, as her digestive system healed, Caitlin regained her energy and her skin cleared. No more stomach upset, no more acne, no more fatigue. Caitlin was healthy in body and spirit and she was discharged from counseling. She graduated from high school with honors and received a scholarship to pursue her college education. We are so grateful to Dr. Fuhrman and nutritional medicine and can't imagine where we would be without this approach."

Gigi Smith
West Milford, New Jersey

FERTILITY

"My husband is a physician, and when he and I first found out about Dr. Fuhrman, we were both very impressed with his depth of knowledge. We converted to the plant-based approach to eating, and we increased our energy levels, lowered our cholesterol, and lost excess weight. Surprisingly, we were then able to conceive our first child. Subsequently, I enjoyed two complication-free pregnancies, which is no small detail since I gave birth at age 39 and 44. That was not a possibility before I started following Dr. Fuhrman's nutritional recommendations.

Our nutrition choices have continued to change our lives and the lives of our children. Because they have always eaten a high-nutrient, plant-based diet, they enjoy fruits and vegetables, and mealtime is a pleasant experience. Neither of them has ever needed antibiotics. They have had no ear infections, allergies, asthma, or persistent childhood illnesses."

Sheila Ott
Greensboro, North Carolina

DEPRESSION

"I suffered for many years going from doctor to doctor, including alternative medicine doctors, and for the most part I got worse. I had severe migraines, depression, and anxiety, and was taking anti-depressants and painkillers. I was gaining weight, becoming lethargic, and had just about given up. Then I started Dr. Fuhrman's plan. Within a few weeks, I was off all medications and losing weight. Amazingly, my headaches disappeared! However, years later I moved away from Dr. Fuhrman, I went through a stressful period and started eating how I used to. I became depressed, anxious and the headaches returned. I went to another doctor who insisted I go back on medication. One day, I was lying in a dark room, coping with a headache and I realized what I needed to do. I pulled out my books, re-started the program, and I am once again free of pain. I learned my lesson: you are what you eat."

Patti Brandt
Tucson, Arizona

ALLERGIES AND ASTHMA

"During spring and summer I was practically the girl in the bubble. My entire life revolved around avoiding exposure to things that would trigger my severe allergies and asthma. I never went outdoors, except long enough to get into my air-conditioned car that was equipped with a pollen filter. Then I started Dr. Fuhrman's plan and my symptoms got less and less severe. I used to associate nice weather with misery and my dangerous medications, but now it's smooth sailing! I feel so free! I can sit next to open windows and have no symptoms and even spend entire days outside. It's amazing: my allergies and asthma are gone!"

Jennifer McCay
Jersey City, New Jersey

FOR DOCTORS ONLY

These limited case studies are only a tiny sampling of the many thousands of lives that have been dramatically changed for the better by adopting this program of high-nutrient eating. For example, so many of my patients have achieved recoveries from lupus that one of them interviewed other patients who had previously suffered from autoimmune diseases and wrote a book about it. Some physicians or skeptics may say, "You claim to have hundreds of documented cases of disease recoveries, but these case histories are not sufficient. You also need medical studies that can corroborate these results. Lots of people can make false claims. How do I know your word is true?"

My response is that I agree that more scientific studies would be helpful, and my office is now involved with four new research trials in 2008. However, some very important research supporting these concepts has been done already, so these cases are not the only evidence that diseases such as high blood pressure, heart and circulatory diseases, diabetes, headaches, and digestive problems can be prevented and resolved via better nutrition. Before getting into the foundation of this program, let's briefly review a small sampling of the scientific evidence that supports this plan and helps explain the science behind the many health transformations that have occurred in people's lives.

As you move forward, keep in mind that there are other diets with some features of *Eat for Health*. Obviously, the scientific evidence over the last 50 years has encouraged many knowledgeable individuals to eat more vegetables and other healthy foods. However, the small nuances that make this program unique make a big difference in the outcome, especially in achieving permanent results. Remember, temporary weight loss is of no benefit. The results must stick forever. *Eat for Health* gets the best results because it has no equal when imploring people to change for the long-term.

One of the features that makes this program work is learning about the healing power of high-nutrient super foods; however, that alone is not unique. *Eat for Health* explains and targets the most critical facets of what makes a diet medicinal. It supplies optimal levels of nutrients, while minimizing excesses and harmful food choices, and does it in a way that makes eating healthfully more pleasurable. It also prevents overeating and removes cravings and food addiction. To truly understand it, you must dive into this book.

Eat For Health and Cardiovascular Disease

The dietary recommendations contained in this book and the elements that make a diet cardio-protective have been tested in multiple studies. The evidence here is overwhelming. Let's first look at the LDL cholesterol lowering effects of various dietary plans, as documented in published medical journal articles.

METHOD	% DECREASE LDL CHOLESTEROL
American Heart Association standard low-fat advice[1]	6%
High protein (Atkins-type)[2]	No significant change
Low-fat vegetarian[3]	16%
High olive oil—Mediterranean[4]	No significant change
Cholesterol-lowering medication (statins)[5]	26%
Eat For Health[6]	33%

Eat for Health puts together many different qualities that make a diet cardio-protective and cholesterol-reducing. It's not just a low-fat or vegetarian way of eating that makes a diet ideal. This eating-style has such dramatic benefits because it is very high in mixed fibers and vegetables and has sterols and other compounds from beans and nuts. This is the only dietary intervention shown to lower cholesterol as effectively as cholesterol-lowering medications. Though the low-fat vegetarian diet did lower LDL cholesterol 16 percent, triglycerides were actually 18.7 percent higher and the LDL/HDL ratio remained unchanged. The results of the study that patterned the recommendations of *Eat for Health* differed in that the LDL cholesterol was more significantly lowered without unfavorable impact on HDL or triglycerides, reflecting sizable improvement in cardiac risk factors. I have hundreds of patients in my medical practice who have witnessed dramatic reductions in their blood lipids, especially LDL cholesterol, without drugs.

Keep in mind that cholesterol lowering does not adequately explain the protective effect of *Eat for Health* in cardiovascular disease since the diet has powerful anti-inflammatory and other beneficial biochemical effects. Even though drugs may lower cholesterol, they cannot be expected to offer the dramatic protection against cardiovascular events that nutritional excellence can. The aggressive use of cholesterol-lowering drugs does not prevent most heart attacks and strokes and does not decrease the risk of fatal strokes.[7] That is, in clinical trials a significant percentage of patients on the best possible statin therapy still experience events; however, lowering cholesterol with nutritional excellence can be expected to offer dramatically more protection and disease reversal compared to drug therapy, without the risk or expense of prescription medication. Consider these articles from the medical community:

1) The effect of a plant-based diet on plasma lipids in hypercholesterolemic adults: a randomized trial. Annals of Internal Medicine (2005).

   This study showed that when two diets have the same amount of fat and saturated fat, it is the one with the higher amount of high-nutrient plant material that gives the best results for cholesterol -lowering and other measurable disease risks. Here is the conclusion without modification:

   "Previous national dietary guidelines primarily emphasized avoiding saturated fat and cholesterol; as a result, the guidelines probably underestimated the potential LDL cholesterol-lowering effect of diet. In this study, emphasis on including nutrient-dense plant-based foods, consistent with recently revised national guidelines, increased the total and LDL cholesterol-lowering effect of a low-fat diet."[8]

2) The combination of high fruit and vegetable and low saturated fat intakes is more protective against mortality in aging men than is either alone: the Baltimore Longitudinal Study of Aging. The Journal of Nutrition (2005).

This study showed that reducing saturated fat intake is helpful in reducing heart disease deaths, but in terms of the potential to reduce death from all causes it is not as effective as diets that are high in fresh vegetables and fruits. The study showed, however, that when there is a low saturated fat intake and a higher intake of vegetables, fruits and beans, the benefits are dramatic. Over an 18 year follow-up of more than 501 initially healthy men, these researchers found that when both parameters were met, men consuming more than five servings of fruits and vegetables per day and getting less than 12 percent of calories from saturated fat were 76 percent less likely to die of heart disease and 31 percent less likely to die from all-cause mortality (meaning all causes of death). The study stated:

"These findings demonstrate that the combination of both behaviors is more protective than either alone, suggesting that their beneficial effects are mediated by different mechanisms."[9]

3) Plant-based foods and prevention of cardiovascular disease: an overview. American Journal of Clinical Nutrition (2003).

The study concluded:

"Evidence from prospective cohort studies indicates that a high consumption of plant-based foods such as fruit and vegetables, nuts, and whole grains is associated with a significantly lower risk of coronary artery disease and stroke. The protective effects of these foods are probably mediated through multiple beneficial nutrients contained in these foods, including antioxidant vitamins, minerals, phytochemicals, fiber, and plant proteins. In dietary practice, healthy plant-based diets do not necessarily have to be low in fat. Instead, these diets should include unsaturated fats as the predominant form of dietary fat such as nuts. Such diets, which also have many other health benefits, deserve more emphasis in dietary recommendations to prevent chronic diseases."[10]

These studies are representative of thousands that illustrate that superior nutrition could have profound effects on each of us and on the collective health of our nation. In my many years of medical practice caring for thousands of patients with advanced and even unstable heart disease, every one of the patients who adopted my nutritional advice for the long-term improved their cardiac condition, and not one has experienced another heart attack. Many physicians using aggressive nutritional interventions for patients with heart disease, including Caldwell Esselstyn, M.D., and Dean Ornish, M.D., have documented similar results. For example, Dr. Esselstyn followed 17 very ill patients with documented, advanced triple-vessel disease on angiography over a 16-year period. The patients recovered, their angina resolved, and they got well. He stated, "In this study, patients become virtually heart-attack proof, which is remarkable since these same patients had experienced 48 cardiac events among them in the eight years prior to joining the study."

The evidence conclusively shows that the national dietary guidelines, and even the improved recommendations of the American Heart Association, do not go far enough to offer people the information necessary for maximizing results. Modern cardiology is focused on drugs and high-tech interventions that do little to extend lifespan. However, for those desiring more than mediocrity and a true protection against heart disease and premature death, there is a clear-cut answer. The most effective and safest way to lower your LDL cholesterol and protect your long-term health is through this health-altering and life-saving approach. The life that is saved could be yours.

Eat for Health and Diabetes

As the number of people with type-two (adult onset) diabetes continues to soar, it is openly recognized that the growing waistline of the modern world is the main cause of this epidemic; however, most physicians, dieticians, and even the American Diabetes Association have virtually given up on weight reduction as the primary treatment for diabetics. Consider this statement from a medical advisory committee: "It is nearly impossible to take very obese people and get them to lose significant weight. So rather than specifying an amount of weight loss, we are targeting getting metabolic control." This is doublespeak for—our recommended diets don't work, so we just give medications and watch patients gradually deteriorate as the diabetes advances. Today, medications are the mainstay of treatment and, unfortunately, most of these medications cause weight gain, worsening the syndrome and making the individual more diabetic. Additionally, the narrow focus on blood-sugar reduction and reliance on medications gives patients a false sense of security because they mistakenly think their somewhat better controlled glucose levels are an indication of restored or improved health. They continue to gain weight following the same dietary habits that originally caused the problem.

It is well accepted that if it were possible for people to stick with weight reduction and high-nutrient eating, that route would be the most successful. Patients with diabetes who successfully lose weight from undergoing gastric bypass surgery typically see their diabetes melt away.[11] Dietary programs that have been successful at affecting weight loss have been dramatically effective for diabetics too, enabling patients to discontinue medications.[12]

Preventing and reversing diabetes is not all about weight loss. The nutritional features of *Eat for Health* have profound effects on improving pancreatic function and lowering insulin resistance over and above what could be accomplished with weight loss alone. The increased fiber, micronutrients, and stool bulk, plus the cholesterol-lowering and anti-inflammatory effects of this eating-style, have dramatic effects on type-II diabetes. Scores of my patients have been able to restore their glucose levels to the normal range without any further need for medications. They have become non-diabetic. Even my thin, type-I, insulin-dependent diabetic patients are typically able to reduce their insulin requirements by almost half and have better glucose control using this high-nutrient eating-style.

Diets high in fiber and vegetables have been consistently shown to be beneficial for diabetic patients and offer considerably better results when compared to the current recommendations of the American Diabetic Association Diet.[13] The dietary advice typically offered to diabetics is not science-based, and it caters to Americans' social and food preferences and food addictions. In contrast, the qualities of an eating-style that maximizes benefits for weight reduction, cardio-protection, and diabetes reversal are described within this book.

Eat for Health and Autoimmune Disease

Working with patients who have autoimmune diseases is one of the most rewarding aspects of my medical practice. Autoimmune and immune-mediated illnesses include diseases such as rheumatoid arthritis, lupus, psoriasis, multiple sclerosis, connective tissue disease, and the inflammatory bowel diseases called ulcerative colitis and Crohn's, but there are also more than 100 clinical syndromes considered autoimmune diseases. Obviously, not every patient with these diseases can make a complete, drug-free recovery; however, the amazing thing is that so many patients can, and do, recover. The recoveries are not limited to recognized autoimmune diseases. I see many patients with pain syndromes without laboratory documentation of autoimmune disease. The ability to achieve substantial improvement, and in many cases complete remission of these supposedly incurable illnesses, is exciting. I have been writing about these success stories for many years, including submissions to medical publications.[14] For the last 20 years, multiple studies have been published in medical journals documenting the effectiveness of high-vegetable diets on autoimmune illnesses.[15] These have been largely ignored by the medical profession and most doctors still deny the effectiveness of nutrition on autoimmune and inflammatory conditions. However, these pages describe the critical features of the eating-style most effective in aiding people suffering with these conditions. Although it is not clear why these studies are quickly forgotten or ignored after their publication, one factor may be that there is no financial incentive for anyone to promote the power of dietary intervention as a medical therapy like pharmaceutical companies do when studies show some efficacy for their products.

CHANGING HOW YOU EAT

In this Phase, which includes Chapters Two through Five, we will unlock many of the fundamental secrets behind creating medical and weight loss changes in your own life. You will learn some of the reasons why a diet rich in vegetables and fruits can create an environment that allows for dramatic weight loss and medical turnarounds, and why, in the first week of using this book, you will immediately begin eating more great-tasting vegetable dishes. You will gain further knowledge about the importance of nutrients and why low-nutrient foods are detrimental.

As you make your way through *Eat for Health*, you will be able to choose your own personal starting point on the road to achieving nutritional excellence and your health transformation. Phase One of Book Two accompanies the information in this section, and supplies you with the menus, recipes, and eating plans you need in order to put this information into action in your life. If you have not done so before then, when you have completed reading Chapter Five, I suggest you review Phase One of Book Two and begin to change your eating patterns. You will soon see excess weight begin to disappear and new levels of health emerge.

CHAPTER TWO

DISCOVERING NEW HEALTH

"I first came to see Dr. Fuhrman because I had high blood pressure and high cholesterol. Even given my medical conditions, I didn't want to give up many of my favorite foods. I was shocked when he told me, 'Then don't.' Instead, he asked me to add food to my diet by eating more vegetables. After the first week, I couldn't believe it: I actually liked eating raw vegetables and making great salad dressings. I added a pound of raw vegetables to my diet each day and lost ten pounds that month—without going on a diet at all! Of course, Dr. Fuhrman was right; I simply did not need to eat so much of the foods I thought I could not live without. After three months, he tricked me. Without making me give up any of my 'favorites,' I chose on my own to eat very little of them. Now, I've lost over 80 pounds and my blood pressure and cholesterol are both perfectly normal."

Bruce Howard
San Francisco, California

To Be Healthy, Eat Healthfully

The thought process behind *Eat for Health* differs from conventional diets. When I first developed my approach to nutritional excellence, I started by asking, "What is the healthiest way to eat?" The method that you will find in this book is the answer that I came to, perfected over the years. The fact that it is also the most effective way to lose weight is a great bonus. Other diets and nutrition plans seem to be based on the premise, "How can we make a popular diet, and what type of gimmick or hook will sell books?" My primary goal in writing and teaching nutritional information has never been popularity or economic success. As a doctor, I have a duty to patients who rely on me for life-saving advice. My goal was to be scientifically accurate and create the eating-style that is most effective for both weight loss and disease reversal, bar none. Nutritional excellence was, and still is, the answer.

One of the most radical adjustments you will have to make in following *Eat for Health* is forgetting what you consider a normal portion size. Typical portions sizes are far too small for this plan. Get ready to discover that eating much larger amounts of the right foods—high-nutrient foods—is the secret to long-term weight loss and great health. While your focus is on increasing your consumption of healthy foods, you may find that you aren't as hungry for the other less healthy foods that you previously relied upon. When you reduce the consumption of these foods is up to you. The sooner that these foods are less present in your diet, the faster you will see dramatic results. Any changes you make that follow this plan will improve your health, weight, and wellness.

The first step towards achieving nutritional excellence in your life is eating healthfully. Eating healthfully is all about eating more healthy foods. It sounds simple, right? It's not a brilliant or original idea, but most people don't understand which foods are truly healthy. Lots of people think a diet designed around pasta, chicken, and olive oil is healthy, but are these actually healthy foods? The answer is no, or at least not in the quantities that the average American consumes them. The reason is because none of those foods are rich in nutrients.

What makes a food healthy is how many nutrients it delivers to your body. In other words, for optimal health we must eat foods that are rich in nutrients, and in particular, foods that deliver the maximum nutrients in each calorie. This can be a strange concept for many people because they are accustomed to judging whether or not a food is healthy by analyzing how many calories, fat grams, or carbohydrates it has. Try to wipe those ingrained ideas from your mind. With this plan, your primary concern will be the nutrients in the foods you eat. However, to eat this way, we must first understand what nutrients are and which foods are richest in them.

Discovering Nutrients

There are two kinds of nutrients: macronutrients and micronutrients. Macronutrients are protein, carbohydrate, and fat. They contain calories. Micronutrients are vitamins, minerals, and phytochemicals and are calorie-free. For ideal health, we need to consume both kinds of nutrients, but the American diet contains too many macronutrients and not enough micronutrients.

MACRONUTRIENTS = FAT, CARBOHYDRATE, AND PROTEIN

CONTAIN CALORIES

SHOULD LIMIT CONSUMPTION

•

MICRONUTRIENTS = VITAMINS, MINERALS, AND PHYTOCHEMICALS

DO NOT CONTAIN CALORIES

SHOULD INCREASE CONSUMPTION

Eating foods that are rich in micronutrients is essential to achieving optimal health. A micronutrient-heavy diet supplies your body with 14 different vitamins, 25 different minerals, and more than 10,000 phytochemicals, which are plant-based chemicals that have profound effects on human cell function and the immune system. Foods that are naturally rich in these nutrients are also rich in fiber and water and are naturally low in calories, meaning they have a low caloric density. These low-calorie, high-nutrient foods provide the ingredients that enable your body's self-healing and self-repairing mechanisms. They are nature's contribution to your health turnaround!

In addition to eating more of these micronutrient-rich foods, we need to eat less of the macronutrients. Every nutritional scientist in the world agrees that moderate caloric restriction slows the aging process, prevents the development of chronic diseases, and extends lifespan. This has been tested in every species of animal, including primates. There is no controversy that Americans are eating themselves to death with too many calories. To change this we must do three things:

1. EAT LESS FAT
2. EAT LESS PROTEIN
3. EAT LESS CARBOHYDRATE

These reductions will be part of our focus, however, this program is not primarily about calorie restriction. Simply trying to reduce calories is called dieting, and dieting doesn't work. The reason this program is so successful is because over time, without even trying or noticing it, you will prefer to eat fewer calories. I know that can sound unlikely. Many people think, "Not me," "My body doesn't work that way," or, "It will be a real struggle for me." However, if you follow the plan, it will happen instinctually. I have seen it happen to hundreds of my patients, with all kinds of different backgrounds and eating histories, and I promise, it can happen for you too.

This is the secret to *Eat for Health*: achieve superior health by eating more nutrient-rich foods and less high-calorie, low-nutrient foods. **It works because the more high-nutrient food you consume, the less low-nutrient food you desire.** Since the desire for these unhealthy foods will naturally diminish, this program is fundamentally about learning how to enjoy eating more high-nutrient food.

Foods are nutrient dense when they contain a high level of micronutrients per calorie. Vegetables win the award for the most nutrient-dense foods on the planet. Therefore, as you move forward in your quest for nutritional excellence, you will eat more and more vegetables. In containing the most nutrients per calorie, vegetables have the most powerful association with protection from heart disease and cancer. This program will show you why a year-round consumption of high-nutrient, plant-based foods is the secret to obtaining superior health and your ideal weight, and I will show you how to use these foods to achieve these results.

So, What Kind of Diet Is This?

Vegetables and other high-nutrient foods are the cornerstones of *Eat for Health*, but this is not a book about becoming a strict vegetarian. Instead, this eating-style is easily described with a word I coined:

NUTRITARIAN
A PERSON WHO HAS A PREFERENCE FOR FOODS AND/OR
AN EATING-STYLE HIGH IN MICRONUTRIENTS.

The nutritarian way to health, longevity, and dieting differentiates itself from flexitarian or vegetarian paths because the label of the eating-style is not defined merely by the amount, frequency, or lack of animal products. Instead, it is defined by the attention to consuming lots of high-nutrient, healthy foods such as green vegetables, berries, and seeds. A nutritarian usually eats fewer animal products than conventional eaters, but may or may not be a vegetarian or vegan. The eating-style is also recognized by the limitation in the consumption of sugar, other sweeteners, white flour, refined oils, and processed foods in general.

My writings in general, and especially *Eat To Live* and this book series, advocate a nutritarian eating-style. It affords many benefits for the individual and society in general by encouraging more people to take better care of their health through dietary improvements. To a degree, most people have some idea that eating better and eating more nutrient-rich foods will benefit them, but they just don't have the information to know what those foods are and to recognize the benefits and obstacles to adopting a healthy diet. So, most likely you already are a nutritarian to some degree and this program is just making it easier for you to crystallize the eating-style you need to strive for to accomplish your goals.

Healthy Food Choices Are at Your Door

For the vast majority of history, a year-round diet that included lots of vegetables and fruits simply wasn't possible. People were limited to foods that were grown locally and seasonally, or a diet based on grains that could be stored for long periods. However, grains are on the lower end of the nutrient-density scale.

Now, it is always growing season somewhere. Improvements in transportation and refrigeration have made it possible to move and store fresh foods around the globe. This has given us year-round access to the healthiest and most nutrient-dense foods on the planet and an unprecedented opportunity to achieve and maintain superior health.

Our understanding of the importance of these foods is also very recent. In the last 50 years there have been over 10,000 experiments showing the value of consuming high-nutrient plant foods. Here are a few critical points from these studies:

- Plants contain three classes of micronutrients that are critical for our health: vitamins, minerals, and phytochemicals. The finding of thousands of phytochemical compounds in natural plant foods is the most significant discovery in nutritional science in this century. We have learned these nutrients are essential for a highly effective immune system and protection from the common diseases of aging.

- A plant-based diet that is rich in colorful vegetables and fruits, such as this one, allows you to eat more food. With so many high-nutrient foods permitted in an unlimited quantity, it makes it easy to eat to fulfillment and still lose weight, without the need to count calories or restrict portions.

- Increasing micronutrients and reducing calories enables the body to produce an assortment of protective health benefits and defy the aging process. In essence, these studies have shown that there is a way to extend life and delay the onset of aging, allowing you to live better and healthier in those extended years.

Fifty years of scientific studies indicate that most diseases seen in modern countries, as well as the leading causes of death, are the result of dietary and lifestyle choices. Scientists have determined that inadequate consumption of plant-derived nutrients results in cellular toxicity, DNA damage, and immune system dysfunction. This in turn leads to increased susceptibility to infections, allergies, and even the development of cancer.

There is a way to eat a diet that helps prevent these health problems and causes you to desire fewer calories. A diet rich in high-nutrient plant foods is the most effective way to reduce your food cravings. As your level of micronutrients increases by consuming greater amounts of high-nutrient foods, your appetite will naturally decrease. The result is that you are healthier and will look and feel young well into your later years. There is no reason for anyone to develop heart disease, strokes, or dementia. To prevent and reverse these and most of the chronic diseases in our modern world, you don't need instructions from a doctor's prescription pad. **The prescription is nutrition.**

The Unavoidable: Unhealthy Food Choices

Many people suffer from medical ailments because they were never taught about their bodies' nutritional requirements. We eat entirely too many low-nutrient foods, which gives us excessive calories without enough nutrients. Our nutrient deprived body then craves more food, and the availability of calorie-rich, low-nutrient foods enables us to eat ourselves to death. A diet based on milk, meats, cheese, pasta, bread, fried foods, and sugar-filled snacks and drinks lays the groundwork for obesity, cancer, heart disease, diabetes, digestive disorders, and autoimmune illnesses.

THESE FOODS ARE HARMFUL IN THREE WAYS:

1) They are high in disease-promoting substances that undermine our health.

2) The more unhealthy foods we eat, the less health-promoting, plant-based foods we will eat.

3) Consuming calories without the presence of antioxidant vitamins and phytochemicals leads to a build-up of waste products in our cells because the body can't remove normal cellular wastes without nutrients. The cells don't have the raw materials needed for optimal or normal function. The lack in some substances and the excess in others age us prematurely and cause disease.

Foods that are refined, including chips, cookies, bread, and pasta lose a dramatic amount of their nutrients in the refinement process. Plus, the process that browns foods and turns a grain into a baked flake or chip creates acrylamides—carcinogens that make these foods even more harmful. These processed foods are not only nutrient-poor, but they also contain elements that contribute to our health problems. They are typically high in salt, chemical food additives, trans fats, MSG, sodium nitrate, and other unhealthy ingredients.

Unrefined plant foods, including vegetables, beans, nuts, seeds, and fruits, are the most nutrient-dense foods, but the average American consumes less than seven percent of his or her calories from those foods. People who eat following the guidelines of Phase Four of *Eat for Health*, however, consume over 90 percent of their calories from these foods. In increasing the amount of nutrient-dense food you consume, you are directly influencing your body's chance to thrive.

CHAPTER THREE

THE POWER OF NUTRIENTS

The Fountain of Youth

All the different types of nutrients are vital to achieving and maintaining optimal health and nutritional excellence; however, phytochemicals hold a special, elite place in the nutritional landscape. When consistently consumed in adequate quantity and variety, phytochemicals become super-nutrients in your body. They work together to detoxify cancer-causing compounds, deactivate free radicals, protect against radiation damage, and enable DNA repair mechanisms.[1] When altered or broken strands of DNA are repaired, it can prevent cancer from developing later in life.

Consuming phytochemicals is not optional. They are essential in human immune-system defenses. Without a wide variety and sufficient amount of phytochemicals from unprocessed plant foods, scientists note that cells age more rapidly and do not retain their innate ability to remove and detoxify waste products and toxic compounds. Low levels of phytochemicals in our modern diet are largely responsible for the common diseases seen with aging, especially cancer and heart disease. These are diseases caused by nutritional ignorance and, in many cases, can be prevented. Approximately 85 percent of our population acquires and eventually dies from heart disease, strokes, and cancer. This is extremely high compared to other populations around the world and at earlier points in human history.

Let's take heart disease as an example. Heart attacks are extremely rare occurrences in populations that eat a diet rich in protective phytochemicals, such as the Okinawans of Japan, but are omnipresent in populations, such as ours, that eat a diet low in protective nutrients.[2] Compelling data from numerous population and interventional studies shows that a natural, plant-based diet rich in antioxidants and phytochemicals will prevent, arrest, and even reverse heart disease.[3] With what we know about heart disease causation, no one needs to die of heart disease today.

Only via nutritional excellence can you address all the invisible, but potentially dangerous, plaque throughout your coronary arteries. Unlike surgery and angioplasty, the dietary approach addressed in this book does not merely treat a small segment of your heart, but rejuvenates all your blood vessels and protects your entire body against heart attacks, strokes, venous thrombosis and pulmonary embolisms, peripheral vascular disease, and vascular dementia. Eating this way is your most valuable insurance policy to secure a longer life, free of medical problems. Thousands of people following my eating-style have reversed their high blood pressure, high cholesterol, diabetes, and heart disease and have been able to discontinue their medications. Nutritional excellence simply made them well when drugs did not. As you can see once again, the most effective prescription is excellent nutrition.

To receive the benefits of nutritional excellence, however, you must actually eat well. Many people believe they can meet all of their nutrient needs by taking supplements. However, supplements can't match or duplicate all the protective, strengthening elements of real fruits and vegetables. There are too many unknown and undiscovered factors in these natural foods. There are more than 10,000 identified phytochemicals, with more being discovered all the time. Only by eating a diet rich in whole foods can we assure ourselves a full symphony of these disease-protecting, anti-aging nutrients. Supplements can be useful in delivering micronutrients found in foods that would be very difficult to incorporate into our diet, such as fatty fish. This is why the word *supplement* is a good one: the pill is supplemental to a healthy diet and cannot take the place of one.

Our bodies were designed to make use of thousands of plant compounds. When these necessary compounds are missing, we might survive because our bodies are adaptable. Without them, we lose our powerful potential for wellness. Chronic diseases often develop, and we are robbed of living to our fullest potential in good physical, emotional, and mental health. Ultimately, we are what we eat. We get the materials to build our cells from our diet because food provides the raw materials that our bodies use to create tissue and to function at a high level. Consumption of healthy foods leads to disease resistance; consumption of unhealthy foods makes us disease-prone.

Eating right enables you to feel your best everyday. You may still get sick from a virus, but your body will be in a far better position to defend itself and make a quick and complete recovery. Optimal nutrition enables us to work better, play better, and maintain our youthful vigor as we age gracefully.

The Equation for Success – Micronutrient Density

As you have seen, the basis of changing your health is nutritional excellence, which means increasing your consumption of micronutrients, and the best way to consume nutrients is through as few calories as possible. This important nutritional concept can be presented by a simple mathematical formula, which I call my health equation.

THE HEALTH EQUATION: $H = N/C$

Your health is dependent on the nutrient-per-calorie density of your diet.

In this discussion, the word nutrient means micronutrients, not macronutrients. Your future health equals nutrient consumption divided by calories. This straightforward mathematical formula is the basis of nutritional science and nutritional healing. For you to be in excellent health your diet must be nutrient-rich, and you must not overeat on calories or macronutrients. The nutrient density in your body's tissues is proportional to the nutrient density of your diet. By choosing foods and designing our diet with this equation in mind, we realize we must seek out and consume more foods with a high nutrient-per-calorie density and less foods with a low nutrient-per-calorie density.

I have ranked the nutrient levels of many common foods in the table below using my Aggregate Nutrient Density Index, or ANDI. This Index assigns a score to a variety of foods based on how many nutrients they deliver to your body in each calorie consumed. Each of the food scores is out of a possible 1,000 based on the nutrients per calorie equation. Since nutritional labels don't give you the information necessary to understand exactly what you are eating, these rankings do the equation for you and give you a sense of what foods yield the highest outcome. That way, you can estimate where your current diet and eating-style fall. Using the ANDI is simple. It is meant to encourage you to eat more foods that have high numbers and eat larger amounts of these foods because the higher the number, and the greater percentage of those foods in your diet, the better your health.

Because phytochemicals are largely unnamed and unmeasured, these ANDI rankings may underestimate the healthful properties of colorful, natural, plant foods compared to processed foods and animal products. One thing we do know about natural foods is that the foods that contain the highest amount of known nutrients are the same foods that contain the most unknown nutrients. So, even though these rankings may not consider the phytochemical number sufficiently, they are still a reasonable measurement of their content and can be very helpful in giving you an understanding of the value of the food around you. The ANDI rankings, along with another food scoring system, based on serving size rather than calories, will be further discussed in Book Two.

NUTRIENT-PER-CALORIE DENSITY SCORES

Mustard Greens, cooked	1000	Green Pepper	258
Watercress, raw	1000	Tomato Sauce	248
Kale, cooked	1000	Artichoke	244
Turnip Greens, cooked	1000	Carrots, raw	240
Collard Greens, cooked	1000	Salsa	236
Bok Choy, cooked	824	Asparagus	234
Spinach, raw	739	Zucchini	222
Spinach, cooked	697	Strawberries	212
Brussels Sprouts	672	Pomegranate Juice	193
Swiss Chard, cooked	670	Tomato, diced	164
Arugula, raw	560	Butternut Squash	159
Radish	554	Plums	158
Bean Sprouts	444	Raspberries	145
Red Pepper	420	Celery	135
Cabbage, raw	420	Mushrooms	134
Romaine	389	Blueberries	130
Broccoli, raw	376	Brazil Nuts	116
Vegetable Juice	367	Iceberg Lettuce	110
Boston Lettuce	353	Orange	109
Carrot Juice	344	Grapefruit	102
Broccoli, cooked	342	Cantaloupe	100
Dandelion Greens, cooked	329	Kiwi	97
Escarole, raw	322	Beets	97
Cauliflower	285	Eggplant	97

Watermelon	91	Honeydew Melon	45
Orange Juice	86	Soy Burgers	45
Tofu	86	Flax Seeds	44
Sweet Potato	84	Brown Rice, cooked	41
Apple	76	Sesame Seeds	41
Peach	73	Flounder/Sole	41
Green Peas	70	Salmon	39
Cherries	68	Sprouted Grain Bread	39
Lentils	68	Avocado	38
Pineapple	64	Swordfish	38
Apricots	64	Shrimp	38
Black Beans	58	Pumpkin Seeds	36
Edamame	58	Canned Tuna, in water	36
Adzuki Beans	56	Skim Milk	36
Kidney Beans	56	Pecans	34
Oats, cooked	53	Soy Milk	33
Mango	51	Deli Turkey Breast	33
Cucumber	50	Tahini Butter	32
Soybeans	48	Barley, cooked	32
Chick Peas	48	Grapes	31
Onions	47	Potato	31
Prunes	47	Cod	31
Pears	46	Banana	30
Sunflower Seeds	46	Walnuts	29
Yellowfin Tuna	46	Pistachios	29

Eggs .28

Chicken Breast 27

Soy Cheese 27

London Broil 26

Plain Yogurt, low-fat 26

Almonds 25

Figs 25

Corn 25

Whole Wheat Bread 25

Feta Cheese 23

Pork Loin 23

Milk Chocolate Bar 21

Quinoa, cooked 21

Ground Beef 20

Whole Milk 20

Dates 19

Peanuts 19

Whole Wheat Pasta, cooked 19

White Pasta, cooked 18

White Bread 18

Bagel, whole grain 18

Peanut Butter 18

Cottage Cheese, low-fat 18

Pizza 17

Popcorn 16

Raisins 16

Cashews 15

McDonalds Cheeseburger 15

Fruit Yogurt, low-fat 14

Pretzels 13

Cashew Butter 13

Bologna 13

White Rice, cooked 12

Potato Chips 11

Saltine Crackers 11

Granola Bars, Chocolate Chip . . .11

Cheddar Cheese 11

Pine Nuts 10

Macadamias 10

American Cheese 10

Vanilla Ice Cream 9

Vanilla Frozen Yogurt 9

Hot Dog, beef 8

McDonalds French Fries 7

Sugar Cookies 5

Cream Cheese 4

Corn Oil 3

Olive Oil 2

Honey 1

Cola 0.5

Nutrient Scoring Method*

Nutrient Data for an equal caloric portion of each food was obtained from Nutritionist Pro software and included: Calcium, Carotenoids: Beta-Carotene, Alpha Carotene, Lutein & Zeaxanthin, Lycopene, Fiber, Folate, Glucosinolates[4] Iron, Magnesium, Vitamin B3 (Niacin), Selenium, Vitamin B1 (Thiamin) Vitamin B2 (Riboflavin), Vitamin B6 (Pyradoxine), Vitamin B12, Vitamin C, Vitamin E, Zinc, plus ORAC score X 2 (Oxygen Radical Absorbance Capacity is a method of measuring the antioxidant or radical scavenging capacity of foods).[5] Nutrient quantities, which are normally in many different measurements (mg, mcg, IU) were converted to a percentage of their RDI so that a common value could be considered for each nutrient. Since there is currently no RDI for Carotenoids, Glucosinolates, or ORAC score, goals were established based on available research and current understanding of the benefits of these factors.[6] The ORAC score was given a factor 2 (as if it were two nutrients) due to the importance of unnamed antioxidant nutrients. The sum of the food's total nutrient value was then multiplied by a fraction to make the highest number equal 1000 and then all other totals multiplied by this same fraction so all food could be compared on a numerical scale of 1 to 1000.

Patent pending

As expected, green vegetables walk away with the gold medal and no other food is even close. No wonder green vegetables have the best association with lower rates of cancer and heart disease. While most people are eating the majority of their caloric intake from the lower end of this table, those that move their consumption higher will dramatically protect their health. The recipes and meal plans in Book Two will help you reach this goal.

During any of the phases of *Eat For Health*, there are some foods that you can eat in unlimited quantities, the *golden foods* in terms of nutrient density and excellence. Memorize the categories below. If you can learn to make your recipes and meals mostly from these categories, you will be maximizing the nutrient-density of your diet, recovering your health if you are currently unhealthy, or preventing yourself from illness and disease in the future.

HIGH-NUTRIENT FOODS THAT CAN BE EATEN IN UNLIMITED QUANTITIES

LEAFY GREEN VEGETABLES
romaine lettuce, leaf lettuces, kale, collards, Swiss chard, cabbage, spinach, bok choy, parsley.

SOLID GREEN VEGETABLES
artichokes, asparagus, broccoli, Brussels sprouts, cabbage, celery, cucumber, kohlrabi, okra, peas, green peppers, snow peas, string beans, zucchini.

NON-GREEN, HIGH-NUTRIENT VEGETABLES
beets, eggplant, mushrooms, onions, tomatoes, peppers, bamboo shoots, water chestnuts, cauliflower, squash, carrots.

BEANS AND LEGUMES *(cooked, canned, or sprouted)*
red kidney beans, adzuki beans, chickpeas, pinto beans, cowpeas, navy beans, cannelloni beans, soybeans, lentils, white beans, lima beans, pigeon peas, black-eyed peas, black beans, split peas.

FRESH FRUITS
apples, apricots, blackberries, blueberries, grapefruit, grapes, kiwis, mangoes, nectarines, all melons, oranges, peaches, pears, persimmons, pineapples, plums, raspberries, strawberries, tangerines.

CHAPTER FOUR

CHANGING THE MODEL

A New American Pyramid

You've gathered by now that the key component to *Eat For Health* is eating more vegetables, fruits, and other nutrient-rich foods. However, these are not the only foods that you eat presently, and they will not be the only foods that you will eat if you follow the eating style I recommend. Let's divide food into three types: animal products, processed foods, and unprocessed plant foods. *Eat For Health* radically reduces both animal products and processed foods in your diet and increases consumption of unprocessed plant foods, the most nutrient-rich foods on the planet.

In a food pyramid, the foods that are consumed in the highest quantity become the base. However, the standard American food pyramid—the source of most Americans' first understanding of health and nutrition—doesn't put nutrient-rich foods on its base. This is one reason why so many Americans are confused about nutrition and plagued by obesity and preventable diseases.

I propose a new pyramid. For superior health, we must eat more nutrient-rich foods and less calorie-rich foods. Therefore, the top of the pyramid, the foods that should be consumed very rarely, will be the foods lowest in nutrients, such as processed foods like chips and cookies. This means that the base of my pyramid is comprised of the nutrient-rich plant foods. These include:

- Green and other low-starch vegetables

- Fresh fruits

- Beans or legumes

- Nuts, seeds, and avocados

- Starchy vegetables (mostly root vegetables)

- Whole grains

When the nutritional landscape of America is shaped by nutrient density as represented in the pyramid below, we will have dramatically extended our healthy life expectancy and will see health care costs plummet.

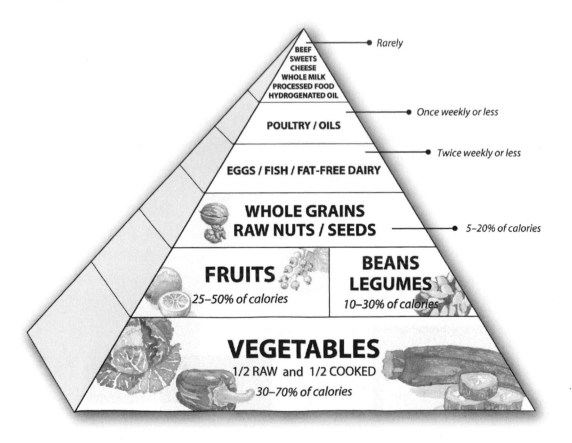

The Dangers of Omission

Our society has evolved to a level of economic sophistication that allows us to eat ourselves to death. A diet centered on milk, cheese, pasta, bread, fried foods, and sugar-filled snacks and drinks, lays the groundwork for obesity, cancer, heart disease, diabetes, and autoimmune illnesses. It is not solely that these foods are harmful; it is also what we are **not** eating that is causing the problem. What we are not eating is enough nutrient-rich foods.

America's Food Consumption Pie

As this chart shows, when you calculate all the calories consumed from the Standard American Diet, you find that the calories coming from phytochemical-rich foods, such as fresh fruit, vegetables, beans, raw nuts, and seeds, is less

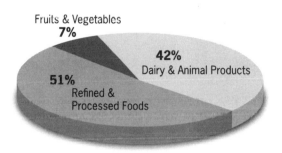

than ten percent of the total caloric intake. This dangerously low intake of unrefined plant foods is what guarantees weakened immunity to disease, frequent illnesses, and a shorter lifespan. We will never win the war on cancer, heart disease, diabetes, autoimmune diseases, and other degenerative illnesses unless we address this deficiency. Though the American diet has spread all over the world, bringing with it heart disease, cancer, and obesity, studies still show that in the populations that eat more fruits and vegetables, the incidences of death from these diseases is dramatically lowered.[1]

Most health authorities today are in agreement that we should add more servings of healthy fruits and vegetables to our diet. I disagree. Thinking about our diet in this fashion doesn't adequately address the problem. Instead of thinking of adding those protective fruits, vegetables, beans, and nuts to our disease-causing diet, **these foods must be the main focus of the diet itself.** This is what makes my eating-style different. Once we understand that concept, then we can add a few servings of foods that are not in this category to the diet each week, and use animal products and grains as condiments or small additions to this naturally, nutrient-rich diet.

Dying from a Diet

Most Americans are not in good health thanks to the standard, low-nutrient diet in this country. The risk of developing high blood pressure, diabetes, heart disease, and cardiovascular-related premature death is extremely high for all people who eat this way. Look at these statistics:

- The lifetime risk for developing hypertension (high blood pressure) is over 90 percent.[2]

- High blood pressure has climbed 30 percent over the past decade.

- Cardiovascular disease (CVD) is an enormous health care burden and is responsible for approximately 40 percent of all U.S. deaths annually.[3]

There's nothing pre-programmed in the human genome that says as people get old they automatically get fat and have high blood pressure. They're getting high blood pressure because their diets are calorie-rich and nutrient-poor. They're eating processed foods and too much salt, and they're avoiding physical exercise. Adding to the problem is that people are given prescription drugs that allow them to continue their disease-causing habits while gaining a false sense of security that they are protected from disease. If you eat like other Americans and don't have a heart attack and die when you are young, you will inevitably develop high blood pressure and then be at high risk for either a heart attack or stroke when you get older. Populations around the world who live and eat differently are found to be free of high blood pressure in their elderly members.[4] These diseases have known nutritional causes, and we never need to suffer from them.

Today, two in five are obese, and the vast majority of Americans are significantly overweight. We are in worse shape today, with heavier bodies and thicker waistlines, than at any time in human history. At the same time, we have learned that our waistlines and our weight are the most critical factors governing our health and lifespan. There is an overwhelming amount of scientific evidence that gives us the knowledge, but people are still dying prematurely and living a poor-quality life plagued by sickness and disability because they are not questioning their current way of doing things. Heart disease, diabetes, and most cancers are preventable, but prevention requires change. It requires learning from our past mistakes and learning new information. It sounds simple, and it can be simple if you have an open mind and if you let knowledge, rather than habits and emotions, guide you.

Learn from Your Elders

Our bodies are designed to live a long, healthy life, free from the common diseases of aging. If water runs over a waterfall and pounds into a rock at high speed, it wears down and eventually splits the rock in two. It was not aging that broke the rock. It was the water that took its toll on it after many thousands of years. Likewise, we develop hardening of the arteries, high blood pressure, heart disease, dementia, and other debilitating conditions from our dietary follies that take their toll over many years of nutritional self-abuse. These common ailments are not the consequence of aging. They are earned.

However, researchers have found that people who exceed 100 years in age are remarkably disease free. Boston and Harvard Scientists recording the New England Centenarian Study (NECS) have been studying many long-lived individuals. Among other factors, they tracked genetics, physical and mental health, and lifestyle habits. They've found that long-lived people generally do not have the age-associated medical conditions that develop and curtail enjoyment of life at an early age. In other words, living healthfully goes hand in hand with living longer. These people, who are now past 100, did not have the advantage of the scientific information that we have today. For the majority of their lives, they did not have access to the healthiest foods. The question is how did they do it, and what skills can we learn from these super seniors?

Without exception, all of the centenarians were not large and certainly not overweight. To achieve your maximum health potential you must manage your weight. **You can literally stretch your lifespan by shrinking your waistline.** Developing a healthy diet and maintaining a stable, lower weight is the most powerful anti-aging weapon in your arsenal. However, we also must consider evidence that nutritional deficiencies have been shown to cause disease and disability. The goal is to maintain a high or adequate nutrient intake and ensure that no deficiencies exist, while making sure we do not consume excess calories. Yet again, the secret is incorporating large amounts of high-nutrient, low-calorie foods into your diet.

When looking at long-lived, elderly people within a society like ours, in which people eat similarly and the average age of death is about 75, we are selecting individuals with favorable genetics. Scientific studies don't tell us much because most of our population eats the standard (disease-causing) diet, so when we look at outcomes it merely reflects genetic influences, not vast differences in the consumption of micronutrients. It would be more revealing if we could look at an entire population that has an average lifespan over the age of 90 and see what the population did to achieve that accomplishment. John Robbins' book, Healthy At 100, reviewed the lifestyles of the longest-lived populations around the globe in recent world history. The top three societies were the Abkhasia in the Caucasus south of Russia, the Vilcabamba in the Andes of South America, and the Hunza in Central Asia. These isolated cultures not only experienced a population with very long average lives, but their elderly also experienced excellent health, free of common diseases seen in our modern world.

The diet in all of these ultra long-lived societies contained at least 90 percent of calories from unrefined foods: high-nutrient fruits, vegetables, beans, nuts, and seeds. Animal products were a much smaller part of the equation, ranging between one and ten percent of calories. These societies all were a physically active people who grew most of their own food locally and ate mostly fresh vegetables and fruits. These healthy societies revealed that, in addition to being slim, there are other important factors that super-seniors share:

- They consumed the majority of calories from fresh produce.

- They had an optimistic outlook on life.

- They maintained a social circle of friends.

- They stayed physically active.

Analyzing the results of these studies in terms of diet, it seems clear that an eating-style that will enable dramatic increases in lifespan and protection against later-life diseases includes:

❶ High-nutrient foods
❷ No excess calories
❸ No nutrient deficiencies

The more nutrients, especially antioxidants and phytochemicals, that you consume and the more variety of each consumed, the better immune function and resistance to disease you earn. You can see these benefits at any age. I have elderly patients that have been coming to see me for more than 10 years, and I have observed blood-pressure and cholesterol readings fall gradually over the 10-year period while these people were following my dietary suggestions and getting older. Rather than seeing the gradual rise in blood pressure and cholesterol with age, I have observed the opposite. After many years, they eventually reach the low systolic blood pressures we commonly see in children. The point is that aging is not the cause of your rise in blood pressure; it is the time spent eating the conventional American diet that takes its toll.

To increase your chances of becoming one of those super-seniors, you should eat lots of whole foods that are naturally rich in protective nutrients. Take advantage of the fresh produce shipped all over the country. Never before in human history has year-round access to such high-quality food been available to such a large population. Eating high-nutrient foods will make it very likely that more people can survive into their hundreds and live healthier than ever before. Even if your genetic potential does not match most of these super-seniors, you can still have the opportunity for a long, healthy life because you can choose to eat high on the nutrient-density line. **Nutrition and other lifestyle factors that you can choose are a more significant determinant of your health than genetics.**

Virtually all disease is the result of the interaction of genetics and modifiable environmental and behavioral factors. Rarely does a single gene variant lead to the development of disease. Common diseases such as cancer, heart disease, and diabetes result from the complex interplay of genes and environment and cannot be classified as only genetic or environmental. The reality is that both genetics and the environment contribute to disease, and the biggest component of environmental causation is diet.

A good example is breast cancer. Less than one percent of women living in rural China get breast cancer, whereas 18 percent of American women eventually suffer with the disease. Yet when Asian women live in America and adopt the richer American diet, which is higher in calories and animal products and lower in vegetables, they earn the same breast cancer rates as other Americans.[5] Genes interact with environmental factors to influence an individual's susceptibility to disease. When these environmental promoters are not present, the disease simply does not exist.

Despite medical advances, 85 percent of Americans will still die from heart disease, cancer, or diabetes. The real key to longevity is not better treatment; it is prevention. By comparison with our sickly nation, people who survive past 100 years are remarkably disease-free. They are generally physically active, independent, and socially connected. They are not the feeble stereotypes that we often associate with getting old. This is not merely about living longer; it is also about staying younger and healthier into your later years, so life can be enjoyed to its fullest. Once you grasp the possibilities, your entire way of thinking will change. You do not have to be a victim. You can experience a long, disease-free life!

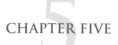

CHAPTER FIVE

PHASE ONE IN PRACTICE

Exercises with Food™

The first step after your study of this Phase is to make some gradual changes in your diet by eating according to the guidelines, menus, and recipes in the Phase One chapters of this book and Book Two. While you are learning about the *Eat For Health* plan and eating the foods and menus in Book Two, I encourage you to do some of my Exercises with Food.™ It is important that you think of these exercises in the same way that you think of going to the gym. When you go to the gym, you can't expect to suddenly build muscle; that takes time. You may not even enjoy going when you first start out. Your purpose is to tear down muscle. Later on, after you have recuperated, your muscle will adapt to the stress and come back stronger. The excitement comes when you see the changes starting to happen. The Exercises with Food™ program works the same way.

The exercises that accompany Phase One strengthen your digestion with natural foods. These foods may seem foreign, and you may not feel the same enjoyment from the food that you are accustomed to. That is ok. The purpose here is to expose you to these new sensations with an exercise mindset. You will 'workout' with food. Many people who taste natural foods for the first time don't enjoy the sensation. These sensations are novel and take time to get used to. Many conclude that the food doesn't taste good. You may simply need more time to get used to their tastes. That is why we have designed these exercises. Like any exercise, you must start small and build up. Don't do too much too fast, but also do your exercises consistently.

The first exercise is to make a bowl of one-half pound of cut up raw vegetables and one-half pound of low-calorie fruits, and eat it slowly each day. This is not that much food. One tomato would fulfill the requirement. You should do this exercise at the same time each day. I recommend doing it in the afternoon before dinner. The important thing is to do the exercise close to mealtime and not when you have a full stomach because you want to feel like eating. Remember not to eat too heavily at lunch, so that you are hungry enough later in the afternoon, before dinner, to eat this extra food. That way, before leaving or when you first getting home from work, you have the desire to eat enough to complete the exercise. The goal of this exercise is to eat a comfortable amount of raw vegetables, including tomatoes, red pepper, carrots, broccoli spears, celery, snow pea pods, and English peas, and fruits including fresh berries, grapefruit, kiwi, and green apple slices. Over time, see if you can comfortably increase the volume of food. That will put you ahead for your Exercises in Phase Two.

After eating all these raw vegetables and fruits, you may decide to eat less at dinner because you feel too full, but let that decision come naturally. Try not to overeat, but don't try to restrict yourself either. Eat the amount that feels comfortable, and try to stop eating before you feel full. **Stop when you're satisfied.** Finding the difference between satisfied and full is an important element of this process.

The second exercise can be done at the same time as the first. While you are eating those fruits and vegetables during the day, chew each mouthful until every piece of food is liquefied. This will take a considerable amount of time and will feel very different from how you are used to eating, but how you eat is very important. Eating slowly is the only way to gain all the nutrients that you want from the food. You can access the full nutrient-load from the food by breaking open every single plant cell. Eating this way will also exercise your jaw and help you develop healthier gums and teeth. Remember: chew, chew, chew.

The most important element of these exercises is performing them every single day. Doing them daily will not only increase your enjoyment of healthy foods, but it will also help you to lose weight. In the beginning, you may continue eating your traditional diet, although you will probably be eating a lot less of it. Over time, you will be more comfortable eliminating your unhealthy food choices and replacing them with healthy alternatives because your palate will desire them. Let this process happen at its own pace. Do not do these exercises instead of eating a meal, especially in this beginning stage. A skill is a developed talent or ability, and being healthy is the result of several skills. The difficulty comes when you try to be proficient in all of those skills at once. Enjoying the taste of healthy food is a skill. Giving up old foods that you love in favor of new foods that you don't like requires multiple skills: abstinence and tolerance. The Exercises with Food™ isolate and target specific skill sets. They will help you avoid the anxiety that many feel when they give up their old way of eating all of a sudden. The method that I have developed is a purposeful and effective way to assist you in your transition to preferring a healthy eating-style.

The Phase One meal plans and recipes in Book Two still include a daily serving of animal products, but this phase has virtually eliminated white flour and refined sugar. The goal is to start you on the road to cooking and preparing foods that are more nutrient dense. Even though you are given a seven-day meal plan, you can eat leftovers for days to stretch out those seven days of menus. You can pick any meals and recipes that you prefer and leave out others. They are all interchangeable, and your eating plan should be flexible.

Phase One Goals
- Have at least three fresh fruits with your breakfast

- Eat a large salad before dinner every night, and chew all of it thoroughly

- Go to the Phase One Menus and enjoy high-nutrient cuisine.

Some people can jump right in and immediately switch to the ideal *Eat For Health* way of eating. I consider the ideal version of this diet to be one that contains at least 90 percent of calories from the healthiest foods; vegetables, fruits, beans, raw nuts and seeds, avocados, and whole grains. For many others, this amount of change may feel too dramatic because they are giving up foods that they love and replacing them with foods that aren't familiar, while adjusting to the physical symptoms of a changing diet at the same time. This modified approach is the one you are learning here and was designed to work in sync with your brain so that you won't feel withdrawal or deprivation.

The focus here is on eating more, not less. The more raw and cooked green vegetables you consume, the less space you will have to eat high-calorie, low-nutrient foods. As the below graphic demonstrates, you will fill a sizeable volume of space in your stomach with a very small number of calories. This will help you comfortably cut the number of calories that you eat each day. This is very much like gastric bypass surgery without the surgery.

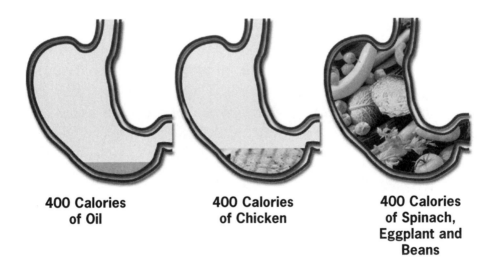

400 Calories of Oil   **400 Calories of Chicken**   **400 Calories of Spinach, Eggplant and Beans**

You will need to adjust the amount of raw vegetables you eat to what your body will comfortably tolerate. If you have uncomfortable gas, cut back a little on raw vegetables and beans. Don't remove these foods, just cut back partially, because the goal is to let the body adjust the timing and secretion of its digestive enzymes and peristalsis to accommodate this healthy, more natural diet-style. You should be able to increase the amount of raw vegetables gradually without a problem. Don't forget to concentrate on chewing better, because that may solve the problem. For some, it takes time for their digestive system to build up the capacity to digest raw, whole foods, especially after eating so little fiber for so long.

While you are enjoying this phase of the program, move forward to Phase Two, and take some time to learn about it while you are living with Phase One. You control the tempo of your progress, but each step is taking you closer to finding excellent health and an ideal weight for your body.

CHANGING HOW YOU THINK

In Chapters Six through Eight, you will learn why changing the way you think about food is an integral part of making the change to a healthier lifestyle work for the long term. You will learn about the psychology associated with food and how to rid yourself of destructive ways of thinking about your diet. Your old behaviors can sabotage your greater desire for health and wellness, so you will learn how to change them. As you have already discovered, increasing the nutrients in your diet and beginning to reduce and eliminate the unhealthy foods you consume are cornerstones of *Eat For Health*. In this phase, you will continue to increase the nutrients you eat while you experiment with broadening your tastes. As you progress through these chapters, review the accompanying section of Book Two and begin to put the lessons into practice through the foods you eat.

6

GET INSIDE YOUR HEAD

"When I was 12, my family moved from Nebraska to Texas. I was miserable after the move and comforted myself with food. Eating for comfort became a familiar pattern, and I struggled with my weight, going on and off diets until I turned 40. At that point, I just gave up trying to be thin. I had had enough failures and struggles. It seemed less stressful to accept being fat forever than to keep failing. I told myself that it was reality, like knowing that I can't reverse the clock and be 20 again. After that, I continued to gain about eight pounds each year until I was over 200 pounds.

Then a friend recommended Dr. Fuhrman's book, *Eat To Live*. I was skeptical. I had tried many other programs, and they were all about meagerness and phony substitutes. I could never resign myself to that. I enjoy tasting food and I like to eat plenty of it, but I read *Eat to Live* and started trying the program slowly, just as Dr. Fuhrman recommends. I was shocked. The program was all about abundance, which was quite a change! What made the difference for me were two main things: the information about how the body uses nutrients, and trying it and seeing that it was not only doable, but also enjoyable.

I thought it would be impossible to give up my favorite foods: pasta, bread, butter, olive oil, and cheese. It was hard at first, but I made the best of it and ate lots of the nutrient-dense foods. I kept eating that way, and, after about six weeks, I realized that I never really missed those foods. It was then that I thought, "This works! I'm eating a lot of food, not feeling deprived and losing weight. I can do this!" For the first time ever, I allowed myself to say, "I'm not going to be fat always. I will be a slim, healthy person!" In my younger years I thought something magical would happen to make me slim. With this plan, I know that it's not magic. I can control it! This is for real and I'm doing it"

Elizabeth Jeffery
Minneapolis, Minnesota

Steps to a Healthful Diet

The American press, diet books, and even most of the scientific research community are thoroughly confused about nutrition and dieting. Almost every article on the topic discusses some magic food, supplement, metabolism booster, or ratio of fat, carbohydrate, and protein that can solve all of your weight problems. Research articles continue to test diets low in fat, high in fat, low in carbohydrates, and high in carbohydrates, and the media continues to report about the successes and failures of these diets. It goes on and on in circles, but trying to micromanage carbohydrate, fat or protein intake will not increase your health and longevity. Worse than that, that sort of dieting encourages temporary fluctuations in calorie intake, leading to non-sustained changes in body weight, often called yo-yo dieting. These diets don't work and are bad for your health because it is not healthy to lose and gain weight over and over. They show once again that diets that don't address nutrient quality do not work.

You must be clear that what you are learning here is different. You must thoroughly understand that it is not some perfect ratio of fat, carbohydrate, or protein that will lead you to your ideal weight and superior health. Rather, what you are learning is scientifically supported information about how nutrients positively influence the body in terms of health, caloric drives, and weight. What you are learning is a new way of living that can improve your quality of life for years to come. Today, we have the knowledge available to maximize nutrition to the point where genetic predispositions will not have the chance to express themselves. The incredible increase in overweight individuals, obesity, diabetes, and heart disease in the last century did not occur because people have changed their genes; it is our toxic food environment. That environment has become so prevalent that it can be difficult to accept the path back to healthful eating with a focus on micronutrients. However, in making this change, you are creating a new environment for yourself, one that allows your body to thrive and maximize its genetic potential. The application of this information to create that environment can allow every person to achieve dramatic increases in healthy life expectancy and longevity.

Unlike trendy diets focused on one aspect of food, following *Eat For Health* requires that you use your mind to absorb this information. You cannot simply change your way of eating without understanding why you're making the change and without changing the way you think about food. To be successful in achieving a healthy diet, you must follow three steps that will revolutionize your health and give you a disease-free life. They are:

1. REPROGRAM YOUR THINKING AND TASTES TO PREFER NUTRIENT-RICH FOODS.

2. REMOVE ADDICTIVE HUNGER SYMPTOMS THAT LEAD TO OVEREATING.

3. LIMIT UNHEALTHY FOODS IN YOUR DAILY DIET.

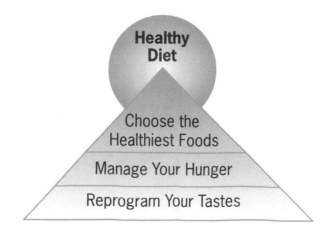

As we discussed in Phase One, as you increase your intake of high-nutrient food, you will desire unhealthy, low-nutrient food less and less. As you progress through this book, Book Two will continue to limit your intake of such foods, including animal products, saturated fat, and processed foods like white flour and sugar. Phase Three will further discuss managing your hunger and ensuring you don't over-consume calories. In this phase, we will focus on how you think about food and how you can reprogram your tastes.

While it is important to understand and think about each of these steps, it's also important to realize that they do not exist independently. We need to eat less fat, protein, and carbohydrates, the only three sources of calories in food. Obviously, we need calories, but we want to make sure that when we do consume them, the fat, protein, and carbohydrates that we choose to eat are all as nutrient-dense as possible. The healthiest way to eat, and the way to make you naturally and automatically desire fewer calories, is to understand the concept of nutrient density and reprogram your tastes. When you understand and try to follow all three steps, you will be amazed how easy it is to achieve your ideal weight and health!

Your Powerful Mind

My book, *Eat To Live*, was written to help the overweight person recover their health and lose that stubborn, excess weight by following the healthiest and most-effective diet. It was not written for the masses, and has limitations for wide acceptance because people's addictive relationships with unhealthy foods are too overwhelming. For many, the *Eat To Live* eating-style is too great a change to accomplish all at once. In *Eat For Health*, the same concept of high-nutrient eating is transformed, using what I have learned since writing *Eat To Live* to make this information more palatable to everyone, and to make it tastier, without compromising the results. What I learned is that for more people to adopt a super healthy eating-style, I need to make more dramatic changes in the way they think before I ask them to change the way they eat.

We are all born with an innate desire to not only survive but to thrive. Somewhere along the line, we have forgotten that fundamental imperative. In our modern society, we have lost touch with our instincts that could lead us into healthful, life-sustaining behaviors. We graduate from elementary school, high school, college, and even graduate school and don't learn the one most important thing we should know: how to live to protect our future health. Consider that 50 percent of our population dies of heart disease and strokes. That number is a tragedy because these are needless and avoidable deaths. The solution is widely available, and yet few avail themselves of it.

For many, even when the information is presented to them, they ignore it because they fear change and loss of pleasure. In a perfect world, people would all live healthfully, get enough sleep, exercise, and eat the high-nutrient diet that would best protect their precious health. This seems almost impossible to do because most people believe that the change would be too hard. For them, my approach seems counterintuitive. It is radically different from what they are used to, and they think it would be too difficult to follow, so they dismiss it. The mountain of supporting scientific evidence is not sufficiently persuasive. They need something more than just cold science to inspire them. Some people are so addicted to their present, dangerous diet that they would prefer death to change. As you continue reading, my goal is to uncover and address all the conscious and subconscious impediments you might face. If you are one of those people who have a hard time with the idea of changing, think you can't do this, or think you will lose pleasure in life if you do, think again. This program was designed just for you.

Conflicting Messages

The principal reason why people struggle with adopting a healthy diet is because they have internal conflict. One part of them wants to be healthy, while another wants to do something that is not healthy, usually something that gives them pleasure in the moment of doing it, like eating a pint of ice cream. In the moment that you hold the carton and spoon in your hands, you want to eat the ice cream. In the larger perspective, you want to be healthy and lead a long, productive life. This book will help you rectify those two desires.

Adopting a healthy lifestyle generally requires change on many levels. Each level is controlled by a different region of the brain, and each level is like a different frequency or radio channel. The information and techniques in this book will train you so that you change on all levels. In other words, you will do work on various aspects of yourself until being healthy and maintaining an ideal weight comes naturally. The goal is to help you to adopt a healthy set of core beliefs and healthy automatic responses so that eventually you will follow a healthy lifestyle without any conscious effort.

That process is not about strengthening your willpower, calorie-counting or any other gimmick. After studying this book, you will no longer need these things. Instead, you will learn the information and practice it in your life until you instinctually prefer eating this way. When you can get the conflicting levels of thought in your brain to work harmoniously together, you will be able to enjoy eating for health. When you achieve that level of internalization, this information will go from being intellectual to being part of your core belief structure.

To achieve permanent success in the health and weight loss arena, we have to consider the complexity of human nature. We are physical, emotional, and social beings. We must consider all of these factors. If not, many people will reject learning more about a health-giving lifestyle, even though they had an interest in gaining more information. This is a physical manifestation of a subconscious process. **Our brains are designed to dim awareness to information that causes us anxiety.** For most people, the idea of overhauling the way they think about food and the way they eat is a source of anxiety. Plus, unhealthy foods are a slow-working poison. Many ailments related to the foods people eat take years to develop, and the only visible issue for most people is their excess weight. Studies have shown that most overweight people routinely underestimate the extent of their obesity and do not see themselves as that overweight. Consequently, it is not too difficult to imagine how so many people can ignore the evidence. They don't see what it has to do with them. This is especially true for people who have low self-esteem.

Addressing Your Self-Worth

The objection of those unwilling to change their diet can sometimes have very little to do with the food. It is often the direct result of low self-esteem, which makes them vulnerable to negative peer pressure, addictions, and emotional over-eating. Some may fear appearing different from others, and they think changing the way they eat will result in a loss of social status. This is a subconscious perception, but some people are unknowingly governed by it. Others overeat to raise dopamine production in the brain, so that they can dull the frustration and pain of life.

As social animals, our brains require certain hormones that are released when we have positive social interaction. Eliminate these interactions and the brain will seek out other ways to produce the hormones and receive stimulatory input. This is why people with strong social ties are far less likely to be drawn into compulsive overeating and other addictive behaviors. Several studies have shown that overeating, like drug and alcohol abuse, leads to dopamine stimulation. For people who are dependent on dopamine surges and who lack the emotional fulfillment that can provide them, consumption of high-calorie foods gives the brain the surge it is looking for. Therefore, they are more compelled to engage in this behavior. Their beliefs about themselves set in motion a chain of chemical events that predisposes them to addictive behaviors. These can make it more difficult to adopt a healthy lifestyle, so it is crucial to identify this and address it to successfully change eating behaviors.

People with low self-esteem do not realize that they are living out a self-fulfilling prophecy. The belief that they are not worthy of attention makes it a reality. We are wired to operate in accordance with our beliefs, and it all happens beyond our awareness. A person who believes that he or she is unworthy will shy away from other people, develop habits that further lower his or her attractiveness to others, and will ultimately reinforce his or her negative beliefs and practices. In doing so, such people often lower their self-perceived social status. Status is an important factor that affects every facet of your life including the way that you eat. It has very little to do with class, economics, or education. It is a combination of what I believe about myself, what you believe about me, and—the most important part for this discussion—what I believe you believe about me. In short, it is a measure of social acceptance. Lower-status people instinctively look to higher-status people for direction, without being aware of it. Lower-status individuals constantly seek acceptance through compliant behaviors, including eating, drinking, smoking, or taking drugs.

Our self-esteem is a core belief; it deeply affects our behaviors in ways that we only barely perceive. Most of us are unable to judge our own status. To get an accurate measurement, we need to examine our automatic behaviors, the things we do without thinking. What are the principle indicators of low status and low self-esteem? A partial list of these includes:

- Conformity or compliance, especially with unhealthy behaviors; a fear of being different

- Social shyness or fear

- Constant deference to others

- Lowered ability to communicate

- Inability to maintain eye contact

- Physical aggressiveness

We need to ask ourselves a series of questions to determine if we are allowing self-degradation to hurt our potential for health and ability to comply with healthy behaviors that will lead us to success and happiness.

- Am I engaged in behaviors that are detrimental to me?

- What are the forces pressuring me to adopt or maintain this behavior?

- Does this behavior increase or diminish my status and self esteem?

- Am I a trendsetter or a trend-follower?

- Am I avoiding a useful behavior because I don't want others to think I am different?

We need to be able to view ourselves in a favorable light and cultivate behaviors and activities that build pride in ourselves in order to challenge these issues. That pride could come from helping others, being understanding of others, having interests that engage us, developing skills, and appreciating value and goodness wherever we see it.

LIST A FEW REASONS YOU HAVE TO BE PROUD OF YOURSELF.

_____

_____

_____

_____

WRITE DOWN THREE THINGS YOU COULD DO TO EXPAND
THE WIDTH OR DEPTH OF YOUR INTERESTS.

_____

_____

_____

Though engaging in these written exercises may not seem to be directly tied to your desire to lose weight and increase your health, I can assure you from years of working with thousands of patients that for lots of people, it is. The key to change is learning social skills so you do not look for bad dietary habits to solve your social problems. Unhealthful behaviors that lead to poor health lower your emotional well-being and further this cycle. You cannot do one without the other. Your beliefs and your diet work hand in hand. It can be helpful to your health and dietary choices to be more confident. If you believe that what you say is worthwhile and attractive to others, this attitude will be transferred to everyone around you, irrespective of how you might actually look. When you have a legitimate reason to believe in yourself, you will care for yourself better and be more inclined to eat right.

We are all prone to follow the direction of the group and most Americans follow a diet that is popular and unhealthy. Could the difficulty some people have of not following the crowd have something to do with resisting change? It is a factor for some people. They want to fit in, and will be uncomfortable eating differently because they believe they will be rejected by their reference group. This perceived loss of status from being different can create a subconscious resistance, presenting another obstacle to change. This is an irrational response; following the crowd does not lead to enhanced status or self-respect and it is unfortunate that an unhealthy lifestyle and a disease-causing diet gains the psychological advantage.

Feeling that you belong within a group of friends, who help you to be a better person and with whom you have something in common, raises your emotional health and self-confidence. It is far easier to change and transition into a healthy lifestyle when you have the support of others doing the same. The more your group embraces and supports you in your efforts to eat healthier and live a health-supporting lifestyle, the easier this becomes. Our American reference group is a nation eating itself to death, committing suicide with knives and forks. Given that, it is helpful to have support when attempting to move away from the dietary norm. If you have a real and tangible social group, you are much less likely to be affected by the artificial ones created by advertisers, marketers, and technology. If you want to get healthy, hang around other healthy people and others striving to be healthy.

Some people will attempt to make you uncomfortable because you are eating healthfully. Your change in behavior may make them uncomfortable because you are forcing them to examine their own unhealthy practices. If you look for approval from someone who is struggling on that issue, you will generally not get a positive response. Don't let this issue subconsciously prevent you from adopting this program. Regardless of the illogical motives of the unconscious mind to save face, you actually lower your social status by letting these forces govern your life's choices.

Eating healthfully and developing the skills to earn and enjoy excellent health may increase your self-esteem, which in turn may help you socially. This is very important as we know from studying the centenarians in Chapter Four that the longest-lived, healthiest people share some common traits, among them, good relationships with other people. The Australian Longitudinal Study of Aging showed that people with good relationships were 22 percent less likely to die over the following decade.[1] Interestingly, close contact with children and relatives had little impact on survival. It was those with the strongest network of friends and acquaintances who were the most likely to survive. Unquestionably developing peers who are also interested in healthy living is a great idea. Forming a support group or even joining our support group on the web can be extremely beneficial and aid in your success. At **www.EatRightAmerica.com**, we have events scheduled where like-minded people can converse, support each other, and even associate and recreate together.

Knowledge Is Key

Even if you have fine self-esteem and a supportive group of people around you, your mind can hold you back from reaching the goals you have for your body. We most often behave in a manner consistent with the way we think. Some of the principles that you are learning as part of this eating-style may seem counterintuitive at first because they do not fit neatly into your prior beliefs. Because we are social animals, ideas seem more believable when more people believe them. They require social proof before they gain general acceptance.

A study published in the European Journal of Clinical Nutrition looked at some of the factors that inhibit people from adopting a healthier, plant-based diet. The study found that the more knowledge subjects obtained about the benefits, the more they had their questions answered, and the more prior myths were shattered with science, then the more likely they were to adapt to a healthy diet and achieve good health.[2] For some, change has to occur in steps, and it has to be at one's own pace. Remember, however, that your willingness to change and your success is proportional to the knowledge you obtain. This is a knowledge-based program. Gaining the knowledge is the most critical factor to enable behavioral changes that will lead to healthier habits.

Some people will decide to ignore the life-enhancing information presented here. That decision is made on a subconscious level. A multitude of diets, nutritional supplements, and even drugs promise weight loss without changing the way you eat. This promise alone is enough to keep people from doing the work to change; it gives our subconscious minds a way out. The subconscious mind is not logical. Many of these diets have been debunked, but that doesn't damage their allure to our subconscious minds where most decisions are made. The good news is that you are not at the mercy of your genes or your subconscious mind, and that you can control your health and weight. Heart diseases, strokes, cancer, dementia, diabetes, allergies, arthritis, and other common illnesses are not predominantly genetic. They are the result of incorrect dietary choices. With knowledge, you can be empowered to make new choices by changing the way that you think.

Ideas have a life of their own. They have inertia. Once they are accepted and popular, they become difficult to displace. Much of what is now widely accepted as nutritional gospel is based on scant evidence, mistaken old notions, bad science, and myths advertised to us by food manufacturers, pharmaceutical companies, and the government. At this point, even scientists and physicians accept the myths and gaps in nutritional information. Many current, popular dietary notions have uncertain origins, but since they have been around a long time, they generally go unquestioned. Once they become this ingrained, they are difficult to change, and they form our cognitive health model. Due to that, when people are presented with new information that falls outside the model, it is difficult to accept.

BELOW ARE SOME COMMONLY HELD NUTRITIONAL BELIEFS
AND THE TRUTHS BEHIND THEM.

Frequent small meals aid weight control

FALSE—Frequent eating has been shown to lead to more calories consumed at the end of the week. In addition, in scientific studies, reduced meal frequency increases the lifespan of both rodents and monkeys, even when the calories consumed each week were the same in the group fed more frequently and the group fed less frequently.[3] The body needs time between meals to finish digesting, because when digestion has ended the body can more effectively detoxify and promote cellular repair. To maximize health, it is not favorable to be constantly eating and digesting food.

Being overweight is due to poor genetics

FALSE—Genetics do play a role in obesity, and people whose parents are obese have a ten-fold increased risk of being obese. However, there are many people with obese parents who are slender and healthy. It is the combination of food choices, inactivity and genetics that determines the likelihood of obesity.[4] Excellent nutrition and a healthy lifestyle will overwhelm genetics and allow even those with a genetic hindrance to achieve a healthy weight.

Milk builds and strengthens bones

FALSE—Medical studies confirm that drinking cow's milk does not lead to stronger bones. In a comprehensive review of all studies of dairy intake and bone strength in 2000, researchers concluded, "the body of scientific evidence appears inadequate to support a recommendation for daily intake of dairy foods to promote bone health in the general US population."[5] Having strong bones is about much more than just calcium. We require vigorous exercise, adequate Vitamin D, and a diet rich in many micronutrients. We will discuss more about this topic in Chapter Fourteen.

Heart disease and dementia are the consequence of aging

FALSE—Interestingly, heart disease as a major cause of disability and death is a recent phenomenon in human history. Heart disease has identifiable causes, and populations whose lifestyle practices do not create these causes do not have heart disease. Cultures around the world eating a healthy, vegetable-rich diet have no recorded heart disease, including hundreds of thousands of rural Chinese.[6] The same diets that are high in animal fats and low in vitamins, minerals, fruits, and green vegetables, also have been shown to be related to the incidence of dementia.[7]

What criteria do you use for accepting new knowledge? Much of the information that I am presenting to you may be difficult to accept because it questions conventional wisdom and accepts only what can be proven with scientific evidence. Learning this material might require you to change your way of thinking and, therefore, change your subconscious cognitive model. It will happen gradually and naturally as you go through the exercises and as your body changes as a result of your new eating patterns.

In the realm of getting healthy, misinformation abounds. Misinformation actually works hand in hand with self-deception. Countless diets advertise that you can eat all of the foods you love and still lose weight. Consequently, why would anyone want to completely revamp his or her diet? It seems like it would be far easier to eat less of something that you love than it would be to switch to eating something that you may not currently like. The problem is that, in practice, this has been proven not to work. Studies have shown that portion-control diets result in significant weight loss that is maintained over five years for less than three people out of 100.[8] These diets are doomed to fail because they do not satisfy our biological need for nutrients, and we continue to crave more calories than we actually require. We overeat because we are unknowingly seeking nutrients. In addition, these diets reinforce the low-nutrient eating that we now know causes most medical problems in modern countries. They are founded on weak science and perpetuate nutritional myths. To become healthy, disease-proof, and permanently thin, you can't escape the necessity of eating large amounts of nutrient-rich, healthy food.

Why We Believe Things That We Know Are Not True

If we were completely rational, all of our decisions would be based squarely on either facts or evidence. But, as we know, we are often not rational, and even people with a complete command of the facts will not make sound decisions.

Consider addicted smokers. They can tell you all of the reasons why smoking is harmful, yet, for reasons they cannot articulate, they simultaneously believe they are better off continuing their addiction. Both their emotional and physical addictions prejudice their judgment, and they make rationalizations to believe something that clearly is not true. Before we judge them, it should be noted that most Americans have heard over and over again that fruits and vegetables are the healthiest foods and are important to eat in larger amounts to protect against heart disease and cancer. Nevertheless, people typically dismiss or diminish the importance of this message. Their subconscious is not comfortable with change, and their subconscious wins.

All of our actions and decisions are governed by our core beliefs. Our core beliefs define the limits of what we will and will not do. Many of you reading this book need to change your core beliefs in order to get healthy. At this point, you know that eating more vegetables has health benefits, but you may not really feel that this life-saving information will give you control of your health destiny, save you from suffering with pain, and add many quality years to your life. Your subconscious mind hasn't accepted it yet. For many people, the partial knowledge that they have acquired is in conflict with their core beliefs. They are unable to accept it, so their awareness of it dims and, with it, the ability to make the change.

Psychologists have long observed that we all subconsciously dim awareness to things that raise our anxiety or make us uncomfortable. Our self-deceptions often lead us into absurd situations that are completely obvious to outside observers. Many people blame the media and big business for the current state of the American diet. The truth, however, is that Americans are self-deceived. There is nothing that prohibits us from choosing healthy foods, but contradictions often arise between the subconscious and rational portions of our minds. For many reading this, there is a contradiction between the way that you enjoy eating and the way of eating that leads to superior health. We are prone to believe what we want to, regardless of the evidence. Our brains are masters at suppressing facts.

Changing our ingrained habits requires that we operate for a period of time with cognitive dissonance. Cognitive dissonance is a psychological term describing the uncomfortable tension that may result from having conflicting thoughts, or from engaging in behavior that conflicts with one's beliefs. It usually results in the filtering of information to disregard new information that conflicts with what one already believes, so as not to disturb one's existing beliefs. When it comes to choosing a new eating-style and developing a new taste preference, cognitive dissonance needs to be recognized so we can get over it and move on. We must face the facts, accept our discomfort, and work through it. Our subconscious might not be comfortable with the changes we are trying to make, but we have to hang in there until the change feels natural. Even your taste preferences can change with time. The first step, of course, is getting started. Learning about this and recognizing it are generally not enough to completely change you. However, they do solve one very big problem: self-deceived people don't recognize that they have a problem. Consequently, they never take the first step needed to change. In recognizing your discomfort, you will be able to acknowledge it and move on, so that you are one step closer to taking control of your health.

CHAPTER SEVEN

MAKE YOUR TASTE YOUR OWN

Healthy Food Doesn't Taste Bad

Long-held beliefs about health and food have created a cognitive model for our society, and that model affects the way we see things and determine what they mean. One of the key principles you need to learn that goes counter to this cognitive model is taste subjectivity. **Your tastes can be changed.** We live in a food-obsessed society. Most people believe that their sense of taste represents something that is particularly unique to them. In recent years, our taste preferences have been hijacked and altered by manufacturers of artificial foods.

Consider the following statement: "*Healthy foods taste bad.*"

Is that true? Inherently, no, but many people in our society would answer yes. If taste were something fixed into our being then this would create quite a problem for those people who want to eat healthfully. Being healthy would require us to eat things that do not taste good. Being healthy, therefore, would be an unnatural and illogical state. However, taste is not fixed in us. It is a learned response. The idea that a food can grow on you is true. Our tastes are the result of our bodies adapting to the foods that we eat on a regular basis. Before the advent of refrigeration and global commerce, we could only eat foods that were grown locally. Notice how people in different regions have different tastes. Are they born with different taste preferences than we are? No, their tastes have simply adapted to the foods in their region.

What does the phrase "healthy foods taste bad" really mean? By itself, the phrase means that people have adapted their taste preferences to prefer unhealthy food. To these people, healthy foods may not taste as good as what they generally eat. However, what if they could change their tastes so that they would not only enjoy, but also prefer the taste of healthy foods? This can happen as you put this program to the test. In the beginning, as you force yourself to eat these healthy foods, you will begin to enjoy them more. As you engage in the Exercises with Food™, practice new recipes, and slowly decrease your intake of processed and other unhealthy foods, you will notice that your taste preferences will change. It's one of the many amazing changes that you will see by making this eating-style an integral part of your lifestyle.

The biggest challenge is changing the way you think. Once that happens, changing your taste preferences will happen naturally. Albert Einstein once said, "We can't solve problems by using the same kind of thinking we used when we created them." This can be applied to your eating habits. The thought process that caused you to gain the excess weight will not be helpful as you try to lose it. You must be willing to let go of the old ideas that no longer serve you and never really did.

Your health and weight are governed by the law of cause and effect. Most people don't fail because of a lack of effort. The most common mistake that prevents people from achieving their goals is that they do the same thing over and over, illogically expecting a different result. They get locked into a single way of looking at things. Taking a different approach requires us to think differently. It requires us to rethink what we consider a healthy diet. For a moment, consider the old definition of the standard diet and the tenets of this eating-style:

EAT FOR HEALTH	STANDARD DIET
Vegetable-based	Grain-based
Lots of beans, nuts, and seeds	Lots of dairy and meats
At least five fresh fruits daily	Lots of refined sweeteners
Oils used sparingly	Oils make up a major caloric load
Animal products two to five times a week	Animal products two to five times a day
Focused on nutrient-dense calories	Focused on nutrient-poor calories

You can see what a major overhaul is required in your way of thinking to strive for a healthy diet. However, with time and focus, eating the *Eat For Health* way will become what your tastes most want to do.

Inflexible Palate Syndrome

This notion that tastes can't be changed is so common that I have given it a name: Inflexible Palate Syndrome. An inflexible palate is one that is believed to not tolerate healthy foods. The assumption on which it is based, prevents people from even starting to change their lives. They believe that they could not benefit from this information because they don't like the taste of healthy food. But remember, our tastes are subjective, learned responses to the foods that we eat on a regular basis. By systematically changing the foods that we eat, we can reprogram our perceived taste responses. By following the exercises throughout this book, and by eating from the menus and recipes in Book Two, you will eradicate this syndrome.

The inflexible palate syndrome is an impediment, and you may discover that you have others regarding your eating-style. An impediment blocks you from achieving a desired goal; however, good health is governed by the law of cause and effect. That states: if you can put into practice the right cause, the desired effect will follow. The underlying habits required to achieve good health are all learnable skills. This is a habit-building, knowledge, and skill-based system. A truly health-supporting diet is the basis for good health, and practicing what you learn in these pages can allow you to achieve and enjoy this eating style.

Reprogram Yourself

As a society, we have programmed ourselves to eat in a way that is unnatural and harmful. We mistakenly prefer the taste of harmful foods. The most natural and healthy way of eating now seems strange, and, as a result, it eludes us. The benefits of eating natural foods, as opposed to processed foods, seem obvious, yet they are lost to many. Here are a few of the common excuses that I hear from patients:

"It takes too much effort and time to prepare fresh food."

"I don't like the taste of fruits and vegetables, so why should I even try?"

"People will think I am strange if I eat this way."

Others who may not have voiced these objections were still thinking these or other negative thoughts. It is the substance of their inner dialogue. This kind of talk is not useful. Its purpose is to prevent you from taking action. It is a type of learned helplessness: you didn't believe you could succeed in the first place. This gives you the rationale for not trying. Right now, resolve to fight those thoughts when they enter your head. Excuses or reasons are not based on facts. They are an opinion formed before adequate knowledge is achieved, and, as you now know, knowledge is the cornerstone to success. Your internal programming and fixed beliefs can have you fail before you even start. A key concept is that our internal programming operates outside of our conscious awareness, yet it influences our thoughts and action.

Psychologists tell us that both these preconceived notions and the inner dialogue that resists change to a preexisting belief are a type of automatic thought. An automatic thought is an unconscious process that determines how we interpret the events of our lives. In many people, these thoughts are negative, pessimistic, and completely illogical. They persist because they operate beyond awareness and because they go completely unquestioned and unchallenged. Our automatic thoughts are the result of our core beliefs, and our core beliefs establish our perceived boundaries of what we can and cannot do.

The key to reprogramming yourself is to select an activity that elicits the desired objective, and then perform this activity habitually. As you continue to perform this activity, your skill will improve, your brain will reprogram to the preferred wiring, and your desired outcome will manifest itself. Your brain is not only flexible and adaptable, but it also will restructure itself to accommodate whatever lifestyle you wish to create. This book and the exercises it contains are designed to cultivate a skill and transform some aspect of your brain and your life. The cumulative result of all of these skills is superior health and your ideal weight. Your brain is ready and willing to make the changes!

For years athletes have done visualization exercises to rehearse their physical specialties completely in their minds. They use their minds to train their bodies. Scientists have discovered how this works. In one study, subjects were instructed to raise their arms while their brains were scanned. They were then instructed to simply think about the act. The limbic brain patterns were identical. The athlete simply learns how to reproduce the same limbic pattern while she is performing it. Similarly, using PET (Photo-Emission Tomography) scan technology, neuroscientists have observed that people with similar lifestyles and circumstances have similarly structured brains. One study was of taxi-cab drivers in London. London streets are very complex. Taxi drivers go through extensive training and are required to know the best route and alternates between any two addresses. When the brains of these taxi drivers were scanned, researchers discovered that they all had unusually large hippocampus regions. The hippocampus is the part of the brain used to handle spatial orientation and navigation. What was even more interesting was that the size of the hippocampus was proportional to the time that the individual had driven the cab. The activity or skill of being able to drive a cab through a complex maze like London caused the hippocampus to continuously grow, long after the period of active study ended.[1] For both athletes and these taxi drivers, practicing their skills changed their brains. For you, practicing how you want to eat will change how your brain works in relation to food.

Just as you cannot expect to develop a perfect tennis swing or learn how to play a musical instrument without both good instruction and a tremendous amount of practice, you cannot hope to transform your health without the ongoing process of putting your new knowledge into action. Moving in the right direction, improving the way you eat, and learning how to handle social situations that encourage bad habits are all part of an ongoing process of healthy change. It is a process that requires time and effort and the ability to learn from mistakes. As the saying goes, practice makes perfect. It is not enough simply to know what to do. You need to do it. You need to practice preparing recipes and eating super-healthful meals until such time as they begin to satisfy your desire for pleasurable eating.

Anyone who has become accomplished at demanding activities, such as sports and music, will tell you that it can be difficult to learn new things. It is not easy to develop new habits, and there is no such thing as a quick shortcut to developing new skills and expertise. To eat healthfully takes practice and perseverance.

When you do something over and over, it creates a pathway in the brain that makes it easier and more comfortable to repeat it again later. That is one reason why it is so hard to change a person with ingrained bad habits. For example, I would rather teach someone who never played tennis before how to properly swing a racket than to try to teach someone who has been playing for years and swings incorrectly. That's why teaching this eating-style to children from an early age would make it much easier to accept. They don't have the bad habits ingrained yet. However, while change is difficult, it is not impossible. What makes it possible is a student's strong desire and motivation to change, his willingness to be uncomfortable, and his determination to work on it until he gets it right. The same thing is true with healthful eating.

The more you make healthful meals, and the more days you link together eating healthful foods, the more your brain will naturally prefer to eat that way. Your taste for healthful foods will develop. It has been shown that a new food needs to be eaten about 15 times for it to become a preferred food. The more days you eat healthfully, the more you will lose your addiction to unhealthful, stimulating substances. With time, you will look forward to—and prefer eating—a diet that is more natural and wholesome.

Your Diet, Your Choice

I sat back and thought about it one day: why do I eat the way I do? So what if I die younger? Why not just enjoy all the processed food our high-tech, modern world has to offer? Why not eat cheeseburgers, fries, soda, and ice cream for lunch, and take my chances with an earlier death? At least I will enjoy the time I am alive, right?

In thinking about it, I noticed that I actually enjoy being a nutritarian and eating my healthy diet. I believe I enjoy the taste of food and get more pleasure from eating than people who live on unhealthy food because I've learned to appreciate tastes, and I know I'm doing something good for myself. I would eat this way anyway, even if there was a slight decrease in the pleasure of eating, but after years of eating like this, I prefer it. The fact that it is healthy is certainly the largest attraction, but health-destroying foods are not enticing to me anymore. However, I am not in jail. I have complete freedom to eat anything I want, and if I occasionally want to eat something unhealthy, I do. But, over the years, I have found that I desire unhealthy foods less and less because over time I have found I do not feel well after eating those foods. The taste was not as pleasurable as I thought it would be compared to other foods that I like that are health-supporting. Also, the great tasting, healthy alternatives to attractive but unhealthy food choices, that I and others have developed, makes it even more easy to choose this diet-style. I do not feel deprived.

So, I eat the way I am advocating you eat. I am not overweight and I am not on a diet. I may not eat perfectly all the time, but I have balanced pleasure and health in my diet so that I am not sacrificing one to have the other. The objective is to have both comfortably married. But, I eat this way for lots of reasons:

- I enjoy this way of eating. It tastes great, and I like to eat lots of food.

- I want control of my health and want complete assurance I will not suddenly have a heart attack or stroke.

- I enjoy living too much. I love sports, travel, entertainment, exercise, my work, and my family, and I want to maintain my youthful vigor and enjoyment of life.

- I feel well eating this way and do not like the way I feel, the way I sleep, my digestion, or my mental energy when I do not eat this way.

- I want to live longer and without medical interference, pain, and unnecessary suffering in my later years.

Eating healthfully is only an option. It is your choice. Each individual has the right to care for their own body as they choose, and some may continue to follow risky behaviors using the rationale that they would rather enjoy life more and live less healthfully or for a shorter time. The fallacy with this way of thinking is the belief that people who smoke, drink, take drugs, or eat dangerous foods are enjoying life more. In fact, they enjoy it less. You might feel temporary pleasure or satisfaction, but toxic habits and rich, disease-causing foods inhibit your ability to get as much pleasure from eating over time. Your taste is lessened or the smoking or drinking loses it thrill, but now you are stuck feeling uncomfortable if you don't continue the habit.

Many people who have adopted my advice and become nutritarians have reversed autoimmune diseases, gotten rid of diabetes, headaches, and heart disease and have been brought back from the brink of death, simply by changing the way they eat. And yet there are a very large number of people who are completely deterred from even attempting this change. Their habits now control them, and they are no longer in total control of their lives. I urge you: don't be one of those people.

CHAPTER EIGHT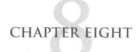

PHASE TWO IN PRACTICE

Exercises With Food™

While eating for health, it is important to continue to practice these Exercises with Food.™ Any of the exercises in any of the phases are appropriate to help you transition to a healthier eating-style. But keep in mind that the focus should be on building up your eating so that you are continually eating more vegetables and fruit until they become the foundation of your diet.

In this phase, we will focus on palate stretching exercises. Instead of stretching your biceps with barbells, you will be stretching your palate and digestive system with a variety of raw and conservatively cooked, natural foods. It's ok if you don't enjoy the taste of these foods at first. When you eat a meal, you expect to like what you are eating. However, when you are exercising it is ok not to like the exercise while you are doing it because you are not exercising for its own sake. You are looking forward to the gain in muscle or endurance that comes afterwards. When first trying something new, we may mistakenly think that we don't like it, when, in fact, we just need more time to get used to it. We can call this exercise "eating without taste expectations". Going through this phase is a necessary step for people who want to create great health.

It is helpful while doing the palate stretching to concentrate on the physical benefits of the foods that you are eating. Habitually stretching your palate will increase your tolerance and enjoyment of healthy foods until, over time, you will prefer their tastes.

The first exercise is to take the half-pound of vegetables and half-pound of fruit that you are eating daily and increase them to one pound each per day. Eating two salads daily—one of vegetables and one of fruit or whatever combination you feel like—is not too much. However, while you add more volume to your diet, also change the types of fruits and vegetables that you are eating. Alternate at least three different fruits and three different vegetables in your diet each week. Also, I encourage you as part of this exercise to try a fruit or vegetable that you rarely eat or have never tried. This is a good opportunity to see the palate stretching in action as you realize that your tastes can change. Grocery stores today have plentiful produce departments that most likely contain something you've not yet discovered. Stretch your palate and your experience in an effort to have a more complete diet.

There Will Be Roadblocks

As we have discussed, there are many impediments on the road to becoming truly healthy. For many people, they can include having low self-esteem, lacking a support group, feeling hesitant about giving up foods, and not wanting to take the time to gain the knowledge necessary for change. Place a score of 1 to 10 on the lines below to indicate the strength of that obstacle in your life:

_____ I don't know if I can learn to like the taste of healthy foods.

_____ I don't know if I can give up unhealthy foods that I like.

_____ I don't know if my family will eat healthy food.

_____ I don't want to eat differently from other people.

_____ I don't know if my friends and relatives will like me eating this way.

_____ I don't know how I will eat in business, traveling, and social situations.

_____ I don't know if I can manage the time to prepare foods like this.

_____ I don't know if I can find enough time to exercise regularly.

_____ I don't know if I can make the time to shop for food.

_____ I don't know if I can learn to cook health food.

_____ I don't like to cook.

_____ I can't afford to spend more money on food than
I do now.

_____ I hear so much conflicting information about nutrition,
I don't know what's true.

_____ Diets never worked for me in the past, so I would
rather not try.

_____ I can't lose weight no matter what I do.

_____ Other roadblock _____

_____ TOTAL OBJECTION SCORE

People can always come up with an excuse why something is too difficult to do. Your subconscious mind may promote this, but a strong desire and commitment to achieve your health and weight goals can silence these objections. With planning and support, you can solve every one of them.

Re-visit this page over the course of following this plan, both when you are feeling comfortable and when you are encountering difficulties. When you are hitting a rough patch, remind yourself that you are in control. You have consciously evaluated the difficulties, and, while that doesn't remove them, it should stop you from using them as a crutch. When you re-visit this page during a comfortable time, score these roadblocks again given how much you've learned by putting the plan into practice in your own life. In doing this, you will see the number decrease, indicating how gaining the knowledge and living the plan is changing the way your thought process works.

Phase Two Performance Goals

- Eat a bowl of vegetable-bean soup or a vegetable-bean casserole or stew daily. This can be from the recipes in Book Two or store-bought.

- Eat one pound of fruit and one pound of vegetables daily. The pound of vegetables can be a mixture of both raw and cooked. Try many of my delicious salad dressings with the raw vegetables.

- Go to the Phase Two Menus in Book Two and continue enjoying more high-nutrient cuisine.

- According to the guidelines in Book Two, further reduce your intake of processed foods and animal products as you increase your intake of fruits and vegetables.

UNDERSTANDING HUNGER

The next three chapters of *Eat For Health* focus on hunger: how to identify true hunger, how to rid yourself of the food addictions that make you think you're hungry when you're not, and why certain foods are particularly problematic and need to be reduced in your diet. You will learn the difference between true hunger and toxic hunger, which is based on addiction to chemically enriched and low-nutrient food. You will also learn about the emotional dynamics needed to be healthy when everyone around you isn't. In coming to understand these issues, you will have taken great steps toward your goals of weight loss and excellent health. Use the recipes and eating guidelines in the accompanying section of Book Two so that when you have mastered this Phase, you can continue your health journey towards even more amazing results. Remember, the pace and extent to which you move forward in this program are up to you. Some people do better changing quickly, and others require more time at a lower phase. Others even may remain at some combination of Phases One and Two for the rest of their lives. However, if you have a significant medical condition, such as diabetes or heart disease, I encourage you to take the plunge into the tasty pleasure of Phase Three now.

CHAPTER NINE

THE COMPLEXITIES OF HUNGER

"When I started following Dr. Fuhrman's plan after I read *Eat To Live*, I learned about the ideas of being addicted to food and feeling the desire to eat too frequently and too much. As I read the description of addiction, I realized that was me exactly. After eating a bagel and yogurt every morning, I could not make it to lunch. I had to have more coffee and some chocolate as a pick-me-up in between meals, otherwise I would develop a mild headache and feel listless. At lunch, a light salad would not do it. I needed the heavy, cheesy dressing to feel fulfilled and normal. I realize now that I was in a vicious cycle of feeling low unless I ate regularly and kept my blood sugar up. It was tough to break the addictions at the beginning, but I followed the plan and made it through until my body didn't feel dependent upon those foods anymore. Now I feel nothing between meals. I feel fine when my blood sugar is low, and I don't even feel like eating then. It is so much more pleasurable to eat when I am really hungry, instead of being driven by my food addictions.

Eight months after beginning the program, I am 60 pounds lighter and still losing, but I am no longer dieting to lose weight. I am content eating pleasurably and healthfully because I feel so much better. In fact, for the first time in years, I actually have the energy to exercise!

Eating this way has also had an effect on my family. My husband changed his way of eating. At first, it was just to support me, but then he began to notice that his eyesight was improving. As he continued to follow the plan, he was able to lower his eyeglass prescription, go off of the cholesterol-lowering drugs that he had been on, and lose 40 pounds. With both of us eating this way, our kids are slimmer, healthier, and learning valuable lessons about food for the rest of their lives."

Robin Rossi
Glendale, Arizona

Moving Forward in Phase Three

As Robin and her husband experienced, if you continue to follow the instructions in this book, you will see remarkable physical changes that are the harbingers of the increasing health your body is experiencing. Depending on your current age and state of health, you will witness a transformation as the pounds melt away and your biological clock is literally turned back. You will be able to physically see that a high-nutrient, lower-calorie diet actively restores and preserves health and a youthful appearance, while a diet low in nutrients and full of empty calories accelerates aging.

At this point on your road to great health, we focus even more on nutrients. Given that, for the remainder of the book, when I refer to nutrients, I will be referring specifically to micronutrients, not macronutrients. As we continue to limit the more low-nutrient foods and increase high-nutrient foods, remember there are foods that you can eat in unlimited quantities because they have extremely high levels of nutrients per calorie. They are:

- All fresh fruit

- All beans and legumes

- All vegetables, except potatoes

As we increase the nutrients, we also reduce the foods that contain empty calories. In the accompanying menus in Book Two you will decrease the amount of animal products down to three servings per week, and most of the oil in your salad dressings will be replaced with avocados and nuts, which are full of important nutrients. With oil, even olive oil, the hidden calories can add up fast, sabotaging your weight loss. Since all oil is 120 calories per tablespoon, it is a substance you want to use in minimal amounts. When you do choose to use oil on your salad or in your cooking, use only a teaspoon per person. It is part of the process of gradually removing more calories from low-nutrient foods and replacing them with more high-nutrient foods.

In this section, we will also discuss sodium and why lowering your intake of it is important to help your body achieve its optimal environment to thrive. As you come to understand this, the menus and recipes that correspond to this phase in Book Two gradually lower your salt use, while the culinary creativity in these recipes delivers great taste without the saltshaker.

The Four Dimensions of Hunger

Though we generically call the feeling that you want or need to eat "hunger," hunger actually has four different dimensions. Many diets fail because they only focus on one of these components—calories. *Eat For Health*, based on the ideas developed in *Eat To Live*, is the only eating style that takes into account all four. Understanding and resolving the drive to overeat must consider and satisfy these dimensions.

1) VOLUME—You must consume an adequate amount of food, and fiber from that food, to physically feel satiated.

2) NUTRIENTS—You must consume enough nutrients in your food for your body to meet its biological need to thrive. Even if you have adequate volume, if it's from low-nutrient food, your body will have a nutrient deficit, and you will feel you require more food.

3) CALORIES—You will be driven to overeat on calories unless the other dimensions of hunger are addressed. The only way to not over-consume calories is to ensure you have enough volume and nutrients so your body can feel satiated.

4) ADDICTIONS—You must break yourself of your addictions to food, which often manifest themselves in ill feelings and cravings. If you don't, your body will not be able to regulate its caloric needs appropriately.

As you can see, each of these dimensions addresses your body's need for food, but none of them exists independently. If one dimension is not tended to, the others will be thrown off. Portion-control diets attempt to limit calories without regard to nutrients or volume. Hunger is never fully satisfied and the undernourished dieter ends up giving in to the overwhelming compulsion to eat more. In Phases One and Two, we discussed the importance of nutrients and calories and how the two work together. Here, we will address the main reason that people eat too much and become overweight: food addiction. Then we will discuss how addressing the other dimensions of hunger can help break those addictions.

Food Addiction Starts the Fat Cycle

When a heavy coffee drinker stops drinking coffee, he feels ill, experiencing headaches and weakness, and even feels nervous and shaky. Fortunately, these symptoms resolve slowly over four to six days. Discomfort after stopping an addictive substance is called withdrawal, and it is significant because it repre-sents detoxification, or a biochemical healing that is accomplished after the substance is withdrawn. It is nearly impossible to cleanse the body of a harmful substance without experiencing the discomfort of withdrawal. Humans have a tendency to want to avoid discomfort, so they continue the toxic habits to avoid the unpleasant withdrawal symptoms. When we discontinue consuming healthy substances, such as broccoli or spinach, we do not experience discomfort. We feel nothing. Only unhealthful, toxic substances are addicting, and, therefore, these are the only substances that cause discomfort when you stop consuming them. Their addictive potential is proportional to their toxicity.

Uncomfortable sensations are very often the signals that repair is under way and the removal of toxins is occurring. Though it may be difficult to adjust to this way of thinking, feeling ill temporarily can be seen as a sign that you are getting well. That cup of coffee may make you feel better temporarily, but any stimulating substance that makes you feel better quickly, or gives you immediate energy, is hurtful, not healthful. Any substance that has that immediate effect is toxic and called a stimulant. Healthy foods do not induce stimulation. When you meet your needs for nutrients and sleep, your body will naturally feel well and fully energized, without the need for stimulation.

The heavy coffee drinker typically feels the worst upon waking up in the morning or when delaying or skipping a meal. The same is true for the many of us who are addicted to toxic foods. The body goes through withdrawal, or detoxification, most strongly when it is not busy digesting food. Eating stops withdrawal because detoxification cannot take place efficiently while food is being consumed and digested. A heavy meal will stop the discomfort, or a cup of coffee will alleviate the symptoms, but the cycle of withdrawal will begin again the minute the caffeine level drops or digestion is finished and the glucose level in the blood starts to go down.

The more you search for fast, temporary relief with a candy bar, a can of soda, or a bag of chips, the more you inhibit the healing, detoxification process. Then, your body becomes more toxic because you gave it more low-nutrient calories. Calories consumed without the accompanying nutrients that aid in their assimilation and metabolism lead to a build-up of toxic substances in the cells that promote cellular aging and disease. Eating low-nutrient calories increases dangerous free-radical activity within the cells and allows for the build-up of cellular waste. These low-nutrient calories also increase other toxic materials in the body, such as Advanced Glycation End Products (AGEs). AGEs affect nearly every type of cell and molecule in the body, and are major factors in aging and age-related chronic diseases. Their production is markedly accelerated in diabetics, and they are believed to play a causative role in the vascular complications of the disease.

AGEs are the result of a chain of chemical reactions and may be formed externally to the body by overcooking foods or inside the body though cellular metabolism. They form at a constant but slow rate in the normal body and accumulate with time, but their formation can be accelerated by your eating habits. Dry cooking methods such as baking, roasting, and broiling cause sugars to combine with proteins to form AGEs, while water-based cooking, such as steaming and boiling, does not. AGEs are highest in burnt and browned foods, such as brown-bread crust, cookies, and brown-basted meats, but these compounds also can build up in cells from the consumption of low-nutrient calories, especially calories from sweets. So, eating both overcooked foods and low-nutrient foods leads to the build-up of AGEs and ages us faster.

When you eat a diet that is based on toxic and addictive foods—such as salt, fried foods, snack foods, and sugary drinks—you not only build up free radicals and AGEs in your cells, but you also set the stage for ill feelings when you are not digesting food. Unhealthy food allows your body to create waste by-products that must be removed by the liver and other organs. Only when digestion ends can the body fully take advantage of the opportunity to circulate and attempt to remove toxins. If the body is constantly digesting, it can't go through this detoxification process effectively.

When detoxification begins, people often feel queasiness or malaise. Eating something restarts digestion and shuts down the detoxification process, making the bad feelings go away. The worse the nutritional quality of your diet, the worse you will feel if you try to stop eating food for a few hours. You will only feel normal while your digestive tract is busy.

Toxic Hunger

Detoxifying your body, after years of eating a poor diet, can be difficult. This is primarily because people often think that, since eating makes them feel better, the symptoms of detoxification they are feeling are actually hunger. This leads to one continuous eating binge all day. It is no wonder that 80 percent of Americans are overweight. Every few hours they are compelled to put something in their mouths. They may feel better temporarily from that chocolate-chip cookie or pretzel, but they never really get rid of the uncomfortable symptoms. This *toxic hunger* will recur whenever digestion ceases, not when an individual is truly hungry and has a biological need for calories. Toxic hunger keeps coming back to haunt you every time your digestive apparatus is no longer busy digesting. Because you feel the desire to eat so frequently, you will become over-weight, and, in the process, your opportunity for a long life and disease-free future is lost.

When our diet contains too much salt, saturated fat, sweets, meat, and cheese, and not enough high-nutrient calories, we are even more likely to experience toxic withdrawal symptoms when digestion comes to an end. Your digestive tract is now actually being overworked almost all the time, you may not feel ill as frequently because these heavy foods take a long time to digest, but when digestion is done, the ill feelings can be quite powerful. The continual eating also prevents the body from adequately self-cleansing. We need a digestive rest between meals so the body can focus on cleaning. Essentially, we become addicted to the toxicity of our diet and are driven to overeat simply to feel normal. Only a heavy meal or continuous eating keeps us comfortable because the minute we stop digesting, the detoxification symptoms begin anew, and we feel uncomfortable again.

Food addiction affects almost all of the American population. Once you address your addictions and use this knowledge to help yourself through the detoxification process, you will be able to more easily, efficiently, and pleasurably address your nutrient and caloric requirements. However, these sensations of *toxic hunger* make it almost impossible to stop a person from consuming too many calories by telling him to reduce portion sizes, cut back on calories, count points, or other typical dieting strategies. You can't easily stop overeating when you are a food addict. You can't expect a person to eat less food when they feel so bad when they do. Unless people are informed, they mistake the withdrawal symptoms they feel for hunger, or claim they have hypo-glycemia and they simply can't help eating too frequently and too much. I call these detoxification symptoms *toxic hunger*. *Toxic hunger* is a physical addiction to an unhealthy, low-micronutrient diet. Its symptoms are generally feelings that we have been taught to interpret as hunger. However, they are actually signs of your body's toxicity.

SYMPTOMS OF TOXIC HUNGER

- Headaches

- Weakness

- Stomach cramping

- Lightheadedness

- Esophageal spasms

- Growling stomach

- Irritability

These uncomfortable symptoms are experienced to different degrees by different individuals. Sugary foods with a high glycemic index fuel these symptoms and the toxic hunger eating frenzy, but consuming too many animal products can do it too. Americans are now accustomed to eating animal products, including beef, chicken, eggs, and cheese, at every meal, but eating such a high quantity of these very high protein foods can overload the liver's ability to eliminate excessive nitrogenous wastes. Our excessive consumption of animal proteins and the elevated amount of waste products puts a stress on your body's detoxification channels and you wind up not feeling well—or detoxifying more—between meals. Some people are more sensitive to this excess nitrogen than others. It is not unusual to find people who are forced to eat a diet rich in protein and animal products. Otherwise, they feel too ill. They must remain on a continual high-protein binge all day. They feel terrible if they try to stop high protein foods or delay eating. These individuals may feel better when eating animal products at regularly spaced intervals and avoiding a light, low-protein meal, but this is the same as drinking more coffee to feel better. It leads to more and more addictive symptoms and they never get better. Just like the caffeine addict, you may have to feel worse for a short time for these symptoms to resolve. Even though the overeating of animal protein causes the problem, the high-protein food also temporarily allows them to feel better and to feel better longer after the meal because high-protein foods take longer to digest.

Eating again to remove those uncomfortable feelings never gets you off the overeating merry-go-round. You can have another cup of coffee or slice of cheese in an attempt to feel better, but it is this cycle that caused you to become overweight and suffer these ill feelings in the first place. To get rid of the toxic hunger symptoms that drive overeating behavior, you may have to feel uncomfortable for a few days to resolve the issue. I often have people make a gradual change in their diet to minimize the discomfort, but eventually as they are able to change the diet more and more, they lose the hypoglycemic symptoms and are able to feel comfortable delaying eating or eating less. This is a necessary first step for them to get back in control of their overeating. Toxic hunger is the main reason people fail on diets. Toxic hunger is a primary cause of obesity and overweight in the modern world. We have adopted a toxic diet, and because of it, we are forced to overeat.

Emotional Addictions

Lots of people are overweight, and most of them know being overweight is not good for their health. Often their friends and family and even their doctors have advised them to lose weight, but they can't. They have tried various diets and simply can't stick with them. As we have seen, many foods are physically addictive, but I want to take a moment to address the emotionally addictive nature of eating as well.

People often overeat for emotional comfort. It can bring fleeting pleasure. Food can be a drug-like outlet to dull the pain and dissatisfaction of life, but, like drug or alcohol use, it is never a good long-term solution. It only winds up complicating things further.

What people of all body weights really want is to feel proud of themselves. Overeating and eating unhealthily cannot achieve this. Packing on additional pounds leads to more guilt and self-hate and, subsequently, more overeating to dull the pain. The solution to this cycle must include more than just food menus and diet plans; an emotional overhaul is needed. Eating behavior has to be replaced with other outlets that build self-esteem and offer comfort in emotionally healthy ways. For many people, these outlets can include feeling proud of yourself for improving your health through exercise, for kindness to others, for doing a job well, for developing a new skill, and for making more choices that will improve your future health. Losing weight can be a powerful encouragement to your self-confidence and to a higher self-esteem. In other words, the more reasons you have to feel good about yourself, the increased likelihood you will succeed in every aspect of your life. Your new attitude must be one that lets go of the idea that you are stuck with your lot in life and that you can't change things. You can.

When you are overweight and you lose weight, you can see it, as can everyone around you. It is a visible representation that you have changed and you have taken back control of your life. You can stop coming up with rationalizations as to why the effort is not worth it, and, instead, you can decide that the rewards are much greater than you ever thought about in the past. But, to get healthy takes considerable focus and effort. You need to plan and put time into this. Of course, it is easier to eat processed and convenient foods and claim you are too busy to squeeze exercise into your schedule, but the effort to do what it takes is well worth it because it will allow you to transform your health and set you free to enjoy a much more pleasurable life. When you first make the commitment to take proper care of yourself and then you put out the effort, you take back control.

These emotional issues are tied into the act of eating for many people, so there is no need to feel alone in experiencing them. If you are someone who experiences these issues, it is helpful to have a friend or a social support so you can share and discuss these topics. It is crucial to address them while also addressing the strong physical addictions that almost every person eating the standard, toxic, American diet has developed. Improving and resolving these addictions is important for weight loss and to increase health and well-being. The remainder of this chapter will discuss some of the most toxic substances that are powerful contributors to food addictions. Food addiction feeds emotional eating behavior, so it becomes nearly impossible to solve overeating problems without addressing the physical factors driving overeating behavior.

The Dangers of Salt

Salt consumption is linked to high blood pressure, blood clots, heart attacks, and stomach cancer. You might be thinking, "Wait a minute. I have low blood pressure. Why do I have to worry about salt?" The answer is that you have low blood pressure for now, but 90 percent of all Americans eventually develop high blood pressure from their high sodium intake earlier in life. Once it is high, it is not so simple to bring it down again with the removal of salt. Instead, that 90 percent winds up on medications to lower it.

Raised blood pressure is a major cause of death in the world and, in most countries, 80 percent of the adult population is at risk. Though 80 percent of the population may not be diagnosed with hypertension, the risks begin well before that point.[1] High blood pressure is mostly the result of a poor diet, lack of exercise, and excessive salt consumption, but according to the Journal of the American College of Cardiology, salt consumption is a significantly bigger risk factor than the other elements.[2] If you already have high blood pressure, eating a low-salt, natural-food diet can remedy your condition and potentially save your life. Even if your blood pressure does not come down with the removal of salt, do not think salt doesn't matter for you. It may take a long time for your body to undo the damage from the many years of excessive salt intake. For those people who have normal blood pressure, removing salt from your diet and following the proper dietary recommendations will mean you won't have to worry about taking medications and you will get more protection against stroke and heart attacks than medications can offer.

In addition to affecting your blood pressure, salt also causes calcium and other trace minerals to be leached from your body, which is a contributory cause of osteoporosis. This is because, as the excess salt is removed via the urine, other minerals such as calcium and magnesium accompany it and are lost as well. If that is not enough, high sodium intake is predictive of increased death from heart attacks. A recent study of adults with pre-hypertension showed that over the 10 to 15 years that the individuals lowered their sodium intake by at least 25 percent, their risk of cardiovascular disease correspondingly fell 25 percent. The conclusion is that consuming a high amount of sodium will put you at a greater risk for heart disease and a shortened life.[3] In another recent study, high sodium intake was predictive of coronary heart disease and mortality from heart attacks, independent of other risk factors, including blood pressure. This means that it is not just about raising blood pressure. More and more direct evidence is emerging that salt is harmful to the heart in other ways, besides its effects on raising blood pressure.[4]

I understand that as you follow this plan, increasing your intake of fruits and vegetables and decreasing your intake of animal products and saturated fats, you may be tempted to ignore the salt factor. You may say, "I'm already making these big changes. I can't deal with taking salt away as well." However, there is another very important reason why we are gradually reducing salt in these menus and recipes. Studies have shown that a certain type of stroke, called a hemorrhagic stroke, increases as heart attacks decrease in a population.

As the consumption of animal products, saturated fat, and processed foods drops down to low levels in a population's diet, heart disease goes to lower and lower levels, reaching less than one percent of the total cause of death. Eating a diet lower in saturated fat and higher in fruits and vegetables dramatically reduces the occurrence of the clots that cause heart disease and embolic strokes. However, hemorrhagic strokes are not caused by atherosclerosis—the buildup of fatty substances in arteries—and the resultant clots. These strokes are caused by a hemorrhage or rupture in a blood vessel wall that has been weakened by years of elevated blood pressure as a result of chronic high salt intake. The weakened wall ruptures and lets blood flow into and damage brain tissue.

Although a low-saturated-fat, vegetarian, or flexitarian diet—a diet that includes the occasional or minimal use of animal products—may markedly reduce the risk for coronary heart disease, diabetes, and many common cancers, the real Achilles heel of the low-animal-fat diet is this increased risk of hemorrhagic stroke at a late age. This is because high-fat animal products contribute to plaque formation called atherosclerosis. Atherosclerosis promotes blood clots that cause heart attacks and embolic strokes. However, this process may also thicken, and therefore protect, the small, fragile blood vessels in the brain from rupturing due to the stress from chronic high blood pressure. When a diet is high in fatty animal products and high in salt, the thickened blood vessel walls caused by the unhealthful, heart-attack-promoting diet actually protect against the occurrence of this more uncommon cause of strokes. In medical studies, higher cholesterol levels are associated with increased risk of other strokes, but lower risk of hemorrhagic strokes.[5]

Admittedly, these types of strokes cause a small percentage of deaths in modern countries, but that is because so many people die prematurely of heart disease or cancer that they literally don't live long enough to experience this detrimental effect of their high-salt way of eating. However, if those who are striving for nutritional excellence, eating natural foods and eating fewer animal products want to maximize their lifespan, it is even more important they avoid a high-salt intake.

Decrease Salt, Increase Taste

Now that you understand why salt must be dramatically lowered in your diet, you may still be questioning how you will do it without eating bland food every day. Part of the answer is that you won't be entirely eliminating sodium. To do that is impossible because all foods, especially vegetables, contain sodium, and this natural sodium adds to their flavor. Up until now, you have probably never noticed this natural sodium because when we over-stimulate the taste buds with too much added salt over a long period of time, our taste receptors can't sense lower levels of salt. Thus, natural, unsalted foods seem to have less flavor. Food then tastes flat without added salt, and you need to add even more salt to almost everything. This is part of the addiction cycle; we build up tolerance for unhealthy substances. The good news, however, is that you can re-train your taste buds to be more sensitive to salt when you decrease its presence in your diet.

Most people consume between 2000 and 8000 milligrams of salt a day. When you get rid of the salt habit, your food may taste bland for a few weeks, but, within a few months, you will find that your taste buds, which were deadened by the overuse of salt, have gradually gained their sensitivity back. You will discover tastes that you never knew existed in natural foods. Even a simple pear or a leaf of lettuce will taste better. Foods that you once enjoyed will now taste too salty.

When we eat a diet low in salt, eventually, our sensitivity to salt and other tastes gets stronger and simple foods begin to have a better flavor. As you eventually get accustomed to a diet that stimulates your salt receptive taste buds less, you can enjoy more flavors in natural foods. This isn't just limited to salt. You will also see the phenomenon at work when eating a simple strawberry or slice of red pepper. Amazingly, your taste buds become stronger when you are off salt and sugar. Try eating some plain romaine lettuce with no dressing on it now. Then eat some after reducing your salt intake for a month. You will be amazed at how much more flavor that plain, unseasoned piece of lettuce has. The bottom line is that once you break your addiction to salt, you likely won't miss it at all, and you will find that food actually has more flavor not less.

Limit Saturated Fat

Just as eating the high salt content in the Standard American Diet will almost certainly cause you to develop high blood pressure, the high saturated fat content in that diet will eventually cause high levels of blood cholesterol, which can then be deposited in plaque on blood vessels. This leads to cardiovascular disease, depresses the immune system, and increases the risk of cancer.[6] Autopsy studies on adult Americans who die in car accidents, unrelated to heart conditions, demonstrate that heart disease is present in the vast majority of American adults. Almost all people over the age of 40 are found to have a significant amount of atherosclerosis in their coronary arteries.[7] The bottom line is if you eat the Standard American Diet or something close to it, you most likely will develop the same diseases—heart disease, high blood pressure, stroke, dementia, and cancer—that most Americans get. You cannot escape from the biological law of cause and effect. If you eat the diet most Americans eat, you will get the diseases most Americans get. Our long-term health is determined by our food choices.

Saturated fat comes from many food sources, including processed foods, meat, cheese, and other animal products. Thousands of scientific research studies demonstrate that saturated fat promotes both heart disease and cancer and powerfully raises cholesterol.[8] It is exceedingly clear that avoiding all fat is not the secret to protecting your heart. **It is avoiding saturated fat, trans fat, and processed oils.**[9] We get heart-healthy fats in their natural, high-antioxidant environment when we eat raw seeds and nuts. Indeed, avocado, nuts, and seeds are rich in fat. They may even contain a small amount of saturated fat, but their consumption is linked to substantial protection against heart disease. But, in the American diet, fats come primarily from meat and dairy, which are saturated, and we compound the problem by the low level of food-derived antioxidants and phytochemicals we ingest.

The table below shows the saturated fat in some common foods. Small amounts of saturated fat are not dangerous, but remember, you should be striving to eat much less saturated fat compared to most other Americans. However, you will see it is possible for people to ingest 30 or even 50 grams of saturated fat each day without thinking too much about it.

SATURATED FAT CONTENT OF COMMON FOODS[10]

	GRAMS OF SATURATED FAT		GRAMS OF SATURATED FAT
Cheddar cheese (4 oz)	24	T-bone steak (6 oz)	18
American processed cheese (4 oz)	24	Braised Lamb (6 oz)	16
Ricotta cheese (one cup)	20	Pork –shoulder (6 oz)	14.5
Swiss cheese (4 oz)	20	Butter (2 tbsp)	14
Chocolate candy semisweet (4 oz)	20	Mozzarella, part skim (4 oz)	12
Cheeseburger large double patty	18	Ricotta cheese part skim (one cup)	12
		Beef-ground-lean (6 oz)	11

SATURATED FAT CONTENT OF COMMON FOODS[10]

	GRAMS OF SATURATED FAT		GRAMS OF SATURATED FAT
Ice cream, Vanilla (one cup) 10		Tuna (6 oz) 2.6	
Chicken fillet sandwich 9		Turkey, white, no skin, (6 oz) 2	
Chicken thigh no skin (6 oz) 5		Almonds 2 oz (48 nuts) 2	
Whole milk 3.3% fat (one cup) . . .5		Sunflower seeds (2 oz) 2	
Plain yogurt 5		Flounder (6 oz) 0.6	
Two eggs 4		Sole (6 oz) 0.6	
Chicken breast (6 oz) 3		Fruits . . . . .negligible	
Salmon (6 oz) 3		Vegetables . . . . .negligible	
Walnuts (2 oz or 24 halves) 3		Beans/Legumes . . . . . . .negligible	
2% Milk (one cup) 3			

Unfortunately, with the entire modern world eating so much low-nutrient food and such a high amount of animal products, it is hard to view a population in which a high percentage of people don't die from incorrect food choices. It is a myth that the French eat lots of cheese and meat, but do not experience heart disease to the same extent that we do. Heart disease, stroke, and cancer still kill the vast majority of French adults, and the percentages in each category are almost identical to the US and other western countries. The average life expectancy in the US is 77.8, and in France it is 79, a negligible difference. The slight difference can be accounted for by the significantly fewer female smokers in France. Keep in mind that small differences in saturated fat intake will not change these statistics much and are not as critical a risk factor as low-vegetable consumption.

While consuming high amounts of saturated fat is clearly dangerous, it is not the whole villain. You still have to keep in mind that consuming the fats that raise your cholesterol is only one of many factors that increases your risk of heart disease, strokes, and dementia. Excessive blood cholesterol is also the result of eating a low-nutrient diet that causes intravascular inflammation and, as a result, heightened cholesterol production due to insufficient fiber, which binds cholesterol in the digestive tract. Your cholesterol level goes up when you don't eat enough vegetables and beans. Saturated fat, and especially trans fat, drives cholesterol higher than simply eating cholesterol does. For example, eggs are high in cholesterol, but eating eggs will not raise your cholesterol as much as eating cheese because cheese is much higher in saturated fat.

Studies in the United States and Europe have established that the incidence of death by coronary heart disease is nearly two-and-a-half times higher for people with the highest 25 percent of blood cholesterol, compared with people with the lowest 25 percent. Yet the coronary heart disease mortality for the same cholesterol levels is only one-third as great in Japan and the Mediterranean.[11] In other words, a person in Scotland with the same blood cholesterol levels as a person in Catalonia, Spain, is eight times more likely to die of coronary heart disease. It is the higher intake of fruits and vegetables in the Mediterranean area that makes the difference.

LDL cholesterol, or bad cholesterol, is the one we want to watch. LDL is very fragile and susceptible to oxidization, which means the fat is partially rotten due to a build up of free radicals. This oxidization is a critical factor in the depositing of plaque on blood vessel walls.[12] Fruits, vegetables, beans, seeds, and nuts are our primary source of antioxidants. Consuming enough of these foods can reduce the negative effects of LDL oxidization. Again, the problem is not just saturated fat. It is this interaction between saturated fat and the low-nutrient environment that makes it a more powerful villain.

A recent study looked at the effects of a diet with more fruits and vegetables combined with a low saturated fat intake. It showed a 76 percent reduction in heart-disease-related deaths for those consuming more than five servings of fruits and vegetables per day and less than 12 percent of calories from saturated fat, compared to those with less vegetation and more saturated fat.[13] Even this small increase in vegetation and mild reduction in saturated fats showed a dramatic reduction in heart-disease-related deaths. Can you imagine the heart protection that would be possible with 10 servings of fruits and vegetables and less than five percent of calories from saturated fat? You simply do not have to develop, suffer from, and die of heart disease if you achieve nutritional excellence.

A Nutritarian is Different Than a Vegetarian

As you know, in living the *Eat For Health* plan, you will become a nutritarian and learn to include more nutrient-rich foods in your diet. A vegetarian or vegan diet that is plant-based also contains a portfolio of natural substances that have various health advantages, including protection against cancer. I am taking the liberty here to use the words vegan and vegetarian interchangeably, but a vegan diet is one that contains no foods of animal product origin whereas a vegetarian diet may contain some dairy. The advantage of a vegetarian (or vegan) diet is that vegetarians are more likely to consume more vegetables, beans, fruit, nuts, and seeds compared to those eating more conventionally, not simply because they are refraining from meat products. Vegans who live on processed cereals, white flour products, rice, white potato, and processed soy products should not be expected to significantly extend their lifespan because their diet cannot be considered nutrient-rich.

Being a nutritarian differs from being a typical vegetarian because the focus on high-nutrient vegetation improves health dramatically, and one can reduce the level of animal products to a safe level without having to exclude them completely. Without considering nutrient density, a vegetarian diet could be just as bad as one that includes a lot of animal products. A vegan diet is an option for excellent health as long as care is taken to eat healthy, nutrient-rich foods. Making animal products the disease-causation villain while filling up on low-nutrient plant foods or processed soy foods will not suffice to achieve health excellence. The reduction in consumption of animal products is only one important feature of this eating-style, not the focal point. Even though you could consider yourself a nutritarian and vegan, the critical issue for disease reduction is not whether one is a strict vegan or not; the issue is the nutrients per calorie of a given diet.

People advocating a meat-based diet may be able to critique a grain and flour-heavy vegan diet as having metabolic deficiencies, but not a diet that is low in animal products and based on nutrient-dense plant foods. This program contains the health benefits of a vegetarian diet, gleaned from the reduction of animal products, without the risks from all those lower-nutrient, higher-glycemic foods such as sugar, French fries and processed grains.

In addition, you do not have to exclude all animal products from your diet to follow this plan and to receive profound benefits to the health of your blood vessels and the rest of your body. You just have to reduce them to safe levels, as demonstrated in the meal plans in Book Two. Humans are primates, and all other primates eat a diet of predominantly natural vegetation. When the great apes eat animal products, it is a very small percentage of their total caloric intake. Likewise, modern medical studies confirm that in order for humans to maximize their potential for a long, disease-free life, they have to keep animal products to a relatively small percentage as well. Animal products are low in micronutrients, contain almost no antioxidants and phytochemicals, and are rich in calories. Thus, they should be limited for health excellence. We want to thrive in our later years, not just survive long enough to reproduce and then deteriorate

The main point here that I want to emphasize, as always, is the benefit of nutritional excellence. In the Standard American Diet, less than five percent of the total caloric intake comes from nutrient-rich foods. This dangerously low intake of unrefined plant foods guarantees a weakened immunity to disease, leading to frequent illnesses and a shorter lifespan. When you eat a truly health-supporting diet, you can expect not only a drop in blood pressure and cholesterol and a reversal of heart disease, but you can also expect that your headaches, constipation, indigestion, and bad breath should all resolve. To achieve this means eating fewer animal products, less processed food, sugar, and flour, and eating more high-nutrient plant foods and exercising. This lifestyle shift is the key to disease protection in general.

The Worst Meat Options

Red meat and processed meats contain more saturated fat and trans fat than other animal products, and, therefore, are poorer food choices. However, the fat issue does not tell the whole story. Scientific studies have documented that red meat has a much more pronounced association with colon cancer and pancreatic cancer compared with other animal products.[14] The consumption of red meat and processed meats on a regular basis more than doubles the risk of some cancers. Even ingesting a small amount of red meat, such as two to three ounces a day, has been shown to significantly increase the risk of cancer.[15] Toxic nitrogenous compounds (called N-nitroso) occur in larger concentrations in red meat and processed meats. Red meat also has high haem (also spelled heme) content. Haem is an iron-carrying protein, and it has been shown to have destructive effects on the cells lining our digestive tract.[16] Processed meat, luncheon meat, barbequed meat, and red meat must not be a regular part of your diet if you are looking to maintain excellent health into your later years of life.

Eating too many animal products and not enough vegetables increases one's risk of cancer. To achieve optimal health, humans require a high exposure to a full symphony of phytochemicals found in unprocessed plant matter. Eating more animal products results in a smaller percentage of calories consumed from high phytochemical vegetation such as seeds, berries, vegetables and beans. Also, since animal products contain no fiber, they remain in the digestive tract longer, slowing digestive transit time and allowing heightened exposure to toxic compounds.

While Book Two will gradually reduce the consumption of animal products in your diet until you're only consuming them two to three times per week, you should certainly avoid processed meat and barbequed meat.

The Detriments of Dairy

Dairy is the food category that contributes the most saturated fat to the American diet. The consumption of cheese has skyrocketed in recent history, and, today, cheese and butter contribute the major load of artery-clogging saturated fat to our diet. As you can see from the saturated fat chart, compared with the same size piece of fowl or fish, cheese could have ten times as much saturated fat.

If there was one food category I could wipe out of the American diet with a magic wand in order to save as many lives from heart attack and cancer as possible, that food category would most likely be the high-fat dairy foods: cheese and butter. The menu plans and recipes in this book do not contain cheese or butter. Animal products that can be included in small amounts are fish, white-meat turkey and chicken, non-fat milk, skim milk, low-fat yogurt, and some eggs, but cheese and butter should be considered special occasion foods only and rarely consumed. Even low-fat versions of cheese are still rich in saturated fat. Part-skim ricotta cheese has over 50 percent of calories from fat, and the majority of that fat is saturated. If you like to include dairy products as part of your limited amount of animal products, only consume non-fat or low-fat dairy.

Beware Processed Foods

Trans fats are extremely dangerous to the body chemistry. Trans fats are man-made fats that are used in processed foods. They are modified vegetable-derived fats that may be even worse than animal-derived saturated fats. They are also called hydrogenated oils, and they are laboratory-designed to have a similar chemical structure as saturated fat. They are solid at room temperature and have adverse health consequences. Like saturated fats, they promote heart disease and cancer.

When you are reading food labels and you see the words "partially hydro-genated" on the box, it is another way of saying trans fat, so avoid it. If you avoid processed food, it is easy to avoid trans fat. These harmful fats are found in crackers, cookies, cakes, frozen foods, and snacks. Most enticing desserts and fried foods contain trans fat, even if they contain no animal products and no cholesterol. Even natural, microwavable popcorn contains trans fats.

In addition to trans fats, the baking of grains and potatoes performed on many processed foods causes browning of the food and the formation of a hard crust, which is rich in acrylamides. In the last five years there has been worldwide alarm in the scientific community after researchers found that many of the foods we eat contain these cancer-causing compounds. Acrylamides form in foods that are browned by being fried, baked, roasted, grilled, or barbequed, but not in those that are steamed, boiled or sautéed in water. Water-based cooking prevents the browning or burning that forms these harmful compounds. Frying and overcooking lead to the highest levels of acrylamides, the highest of which are found in fried chips, such as potato chips, French fries, and sugar-coated breakfast cereals.

Even though these chemicals have been shown to be potent carcinogens in animal models, so many acrylamides are consumed in the modern world that good research documenting the extent of the cancer risk in humans does not yet exist. This topic is still being actively investigated in many different countries, but the risk is difficult to estimate because baked, browned, and fried foods are so ubiquitous in Western diets.

European governments permit far less acrylamides in packaged foods than the U.S. and, they have been advising food manufacturers to reduce them. Cereals and processed foods manufactured in the United States are not under such restraints and have much higher acrylamide levels. Since the same browned and hard-baked products are rich sources of the Advanced Glycation End Products previously discussed, there are plenty of reasons to minimize or avoid these foods in your diet.

The Caffeine Drug

As you know, caffeine is one of the most addictive substances in a standard diet, and there is some research that indicates that excessive consumption of caffeinated beverages may pose a risk to your well-being. Coffee, however, does contain chlorogenic acid, a phenol with strong antioxidant activity which may benefit people who hardly eat vegetables. So in spite of hundreds of studies showing slight increased risk of certain diseases such as osteoporosis and heart disease, there are also studies that show certain health benefits from coffee.[17] Overall, both the risks and the supposed benefits are marginal either way. One or two cups of coffee per day is not likely to cause significant disease risks.

Besides the slightly increased risk of osteoporosis or heart disease, there are other problems. Caffeine is a stimulant, so it enables you to more comfortably get by on less sleep, and inadequate sleep promotes disease and premature aging.[18] Drinking coffee also boosts estrogen levels, which worsens problems like endometriosis, breast pain, and menstrual disorders. Increased estrogen levels are also linked to higher risk of breast cancer.[19] Overall, it is difficult to discern the precise risks from heavy coffee drinking because most people who drink lots of coffee participate in lots of other unhealthy behaviors as well.

My main objection to drinking coffee is that it may promote more frequent eating and a higher calorie intake in some people, so eliminating your caffeine intake may help you lose weight. Coffee drinkers—and tea and cola drinkers—are drawn to eat more frequently then necessary. They eat extra meals and snacks because they mistake unpleasant caffeine withdrawal symptoms with hunger. They can't tell the difference between true hunger and the discomfort that accompanies caffeine withdrawal.

In essence, coffee is mostly like a drug, not a food. In spite of the presence of some beneficial antioxidants it also has some negative effects and withdrawal symptoms that may fuel drinking and eating behavior. Like most drugs, it could have some minor benefits, but its toxic effects and resultant risks likely overwhelm those minor advantages. It is best if we aim to meet our nutritional needs with as little exposure to stimulating substances as possible. This program will work more effectively if you are able to gradually reduce and eventually eliminate coffee and other caffeine-containing substances, as you will be better connected to your body's true hunger signals.

Coping with the Toxic Change

It takes time to be comfortable with the changes in your life. It is not unusual to feel physically uncomfortable as you detoxify in the process of making over your body chemistry with a healthful diet. The more stimulating or harmful your prior habits, the worse you feel when you stop them. When breaking your addiction to salt, meat, dairy, saturated fat, processed foods and other substances, you might feel headachy, fatigued, or even a little itchy or ill, but the good news is these symptoms rarely last longer than a week or two. However, if you are making the changes to nutritional excellence gradually, as modeled in this book, uncomfortable symptoms should be minimized.

Some people are so addicted to stimulating food, sugary sweets, and overeating, they may even feel depressed when they don't indulge. For example, cheese, salt, and chocolate are all addictive, and it takes a prolonged period of abstinence to beat these addictions. Sugar and caffeine, especially when mixed together, are highly addictive and create a significant amount of discomfort when stopping. Sugar withdrawal symptoms have been demonstrated to be similar to withdrawal symptoms from opiates, including anxiety and tremors.[20] I have observed many individuals with a history of severe chronic headaches, who were on drugs for headache suppression, develop fever, backaches, diarrhea, and other severe detoxification symptoms when stopping medications that contain caffeine, such as Excedrin, Fiorinal and Fioricet. Fortunately, their suffering was short-lived. Through high-nutrient eating, these individuals have been able to make dramatic recoveries.

High-nutrient eating was crucial for this result. Toxic wastes build up in our tissues, and we are unable to remove them unless high-levels of phytochemicals are present and the intake of toxins is stopped. You must allow this detoxification to occur. An important hurdle to achieving your ideal weight and excellent health is getting rid of your addictions. After that occurs, you may feel like you have been freed from prison and will find it easier to move forward with the program and be one step closer to truly eating for health.

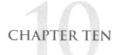

CHAPTER TEN

TRUE HUNGER

Hunger Can Help You Be Healthy

Eat For Health can set you free from your food addictions and allow you to lose your *toxic hunger*. The food cravings will end and you will be able to stop overeating. Then, you will be back in contact with *true hunger*. When you achieve that, you will be able to accurately sense the calories you need to maintain your health and lean body.

I want to reiterate that as you adopt a high-nutrient eating-style by eating lots of healthy foods, it is common to go through an adjustment period in which you experience fatigue, weakness, lightheadedness, headaches, gas, and other mild symptoms. This generally lasts less than a week. Don't panic or buy into the myth that to get relief you need more heavy or stimulating foods, such as high-protein foods, sweets, or coffee.

The feelings associated with these symptoms are *not* how true hunger feels. It is our unhealthy tendency to eat without experiencing true hunger that has caused us to become overweight in the first place. To have become overweight, a person's food cravings, recreational eating, and other addictive drives that induce eating had to come into play. Poor nutrition causes these cravings, and nutritional excellence helps normalize or remove them. You will no longer need to overeat when you eat healthfully.

True hunger is not felt in the stomach or the head. When you eat healthfully and don't overeat, you eventually are able to sense true hunger and accurately assess your caloric needs. Once your body attains a certain level of better health, you will begin to feel the difference between true hunger and just eating due to desire, boredom, stress, or withdrawal symptoms. The best way to understand true hunger is to experience it for yourself. It has three primary characteristics:

❶ A SENSATION IN YOUR THROAT
❷ INCREASED SALIVATION
❸ A DRAMATICALLY-HEIGHTENED TASTE SENSATION

Being in touch with true hunger will help you reach your ideal weight, and also feel well whether you eat, delay eating, or skip a meal. Almost all of my patients who suffered with headaches and so-called "hypoglycemia" have gotten well permanently following my nutritional recommendations.

How True Hunger Works
In real life, people generally snack between meals to satisfy toxic hunger and food cravings, or they consume empty calories and toxic food while eating for recreational purposes. Recreational eating is eating because you are in a social setting or simply because there is food around you. Recreational eating can still occur without satisfying toxic hunger or true hunger. Sometimes people—including me—just enjoy eating good-tasting food when it is offered, even though we are not feeling any symptoms directing us to eat. When most people eat in this way, they do it with junk food, not healthy, natural foods. The way we can reduce recreational eating is by experiencing how much more enjoyable it is to eat when we are really hungry. Then we find that the food tastes much better. This heightened taste sensation that accompanies true hunger gives us terrific feedback to inhibit overeating behavior so we can actually get more pleasure out of our diet. Delaying eating, to the point when true hunger is experienced, makes even ordinary foods taste great and extraordinary foods taste even better.

In our present toxic food environment, humans have lost the ability to connect with the body signals that tell them how much food they actually need. They have become slaves to withdrawal symptoms and eat all day long when there is no biological need for calories. Nature had a different plan. In an environment of healthy food choices, we would not feel any signals that it is time to eat after a meal until the hormonal and neurological messengers indicated the glycogen reserves in the liver were decreased and lean body mass would soon be used as an energy source. Your body has the beautifully orchestrated ability to give you the precise signals to tell you exactly how much to eat to maintain an ideal weight for your long-term health. These signals are what I call *true hunger*. This name also differentiates it from toxic hunger, which is what everyone else, including some medical textbooks, refers to simply as hunger. Most Americans have not felt true hunger since they were toddlers.

Feeding ourselves to satisfy true hunger cannot cause weight gain, and, if we only ate when truly hungry, it would be almost impossible for anyone to become overweight. True hunger is a signal for us to eat to maintain our muscle mass. Eating to satisfy true hunger does not put fat on our body. Excessive fat stores are developed only from eating outside of our body's true hunger demands.

When you get back in touch with true hunger, you will instinctually know how much to eat. When you exercise more, you will get more and more frequent hunger; when you exercise less, you will get much less hunger. Your body will become a precise calorie-measuring computer and steer you in the right direction just from eating the amount that feels right and makes food taste best. In order to achieve an ideal weight and consume the exact amount of calories to maintain a lean body mass that will prolong life, you must get rid of toxic hunger and get back in touch with true hunger. Eat when hungry, and don't eat when not hungry and you will never have to diet or be overweight again. You do not have to carry around a calculator and a scale to figure out how much to eat. A healthy body will give you the correct signals.

So, in order to achieve superior health, maximize your longevity potential and achieve your ideal weight, you have to get healthy enough to get back in touch with true hunger and rid yourself of toxic hunger. To accomplish this, we must obtain high levels of micronutrients in our tissues in order to normalize our cellular detoxification and get the low-nutrient, fake foods out of our diets.

It is not very uncomfortable to feel true hunger. True hunger does not involve your stomach fluttering or cramping. When you feel it, you know it is a normal reaction that signals a need for food. It signals that the body is physiologically ready to digest, and the digestive glands have regained their capacity to secrete enzymes appropriately. It makes food taste much better when you eat, and it makes eating much more pleasurable. People are consistently amazed at how good the simplest foods can taste when they are truly hungry.

True hunger requires no special food to satisfy it. It is satisfied by eating almost anything. You can't crave some particular food and call it hunger. A craving by definition is an addictive drive, not something felt by a person who is not an addict. Remember, almost all Americans are addicted to their toxic habits. A disease-causing diet is addicting. A health-supporting diet is not.

Getting Enough Volume

Our hunger drive craves volume. A key skill that you are developing for your health is the ability to eat large volumes of raw and cooked, high-nutrient, low-calorie foods every single day. This means eating lots of vegetables. It may be helpful to look again at the image of three stomachs from Chapter Five. Each is filled with the same amount of calories, but one with oil, one with chicken, and one with vegetables. The stomachs with the oil and chicken have a great deal of room in them, room that can enable you to easily overeat on calories. That's why filling your stomach with high-nutrient foods is so important to acquiring and maintaining a healthy weight. This leads us to a counterintuitive, but crucial rule: to lose more weight, and for better health, eat more high-volume, low-calorie foods. To lose more, eat more.

When you are actively trying to lose weight, you should strive to satisfy your volume requirements first, before addressing the other dimensions of hunger. This may feel strange at first because you may not immediately feel satisfied by the higher volume of food. This is because you are accustomed to eating large quantities of high-calorie foods that cause a dopamine rush, a rush that low-calorie foods don't deliver. However, your body will adjust, be less dependent on the dopamine surge in the brain, and will gradually become more and more satisfied with fewer calories. Give yourself time, and use the knowledge you have gained. Striving to fulfill your body's volume and nutrient requirements can help you resolve food cravings and your toxic hunger.

The trick to get you to desire fewer calories faster is to eat lots of these high-volume, high-nutrient foods. You are already familiar with these, but many of the foods that you have been incorporating into your diet because of their nutrient values are also great tools in meeting your volume requirements. They include:

RAW VEGETABLES—lettuce, tomatoes, peppers, celery, anise, snow pea pods, carrots, beets, cucumbers, water chestnuts, red cabbage, onion

MOST FRESH FRUITS—melons, oranges, grapefruits, apples, kiwis, berries, papaya

COOKED GREEN VEGETABLES—Brussels sprouts, string beans, artichokes, asparagus, broccoli, Chinese cabbage, bok choy

OTHER NON-GREEN VEGETABLES—mushrooms, eggplant, sun-dried tomatoes, onions, bean sprouts, cauliflower, spaghetti squash

Especially on holidays and days when you know that you will be around a lot of unhealthy foods, pre-fill with these high-nutrient, low-calorie foods. Never go to a party or event with an empty stomach. Eat a large salad with assorted raw vegetables and a bowl of vegetable soup before going to the places that may tempt your desire to eat unhealthily. Being healthy is about being in control. You must control your hunger, and the more low-calorie, high volume foods you consume, the less high-calorie food you will be able to eat. When you increase these super-healthy foods in your diet, you will feel less temptation, and you will be in control of your food cravings and appetite.

The Good Fats

Nuts and seeds are some of nature's ideal foods for humans and the best way for us to get our healthy fats. They can satiate true hunger better than oils because they are rich in critical nutrients and fibers and have one-quarter the calories of an equal amount of oil. They should be part of your healthy eating-style. Many people perceive raw nuts as high-fat, high-calorie foods that should be avoided or consumed in only token amounts. The important role of raw nuts and seeds in the American diet has been almost completely ignored by nutritional advisers, and their absence is a huge flaw in American cuisine. The results of recent research have changed this perception completely. Today, more and more researchers are finally aware that it is not fat in general that is the villain, but saturated fat, trans fat, and fats consumed in a processed form. Fats from avocado, raw nuts, and seeds are rich in antioxidants and phytochemicals that not only offer unique health benefits, but also maintain the freshness of the food, preventing rancidity of the fat within.

Recent evidence shows that the frequent consumption of nuts is strongly protective against heart disease. It has been shown that people eating nuts daily, or more than once a day, had a 59 percent lower risk of fatal coronary heart disease.[1] In addition, several clinical studies have observed beneficial effects of diets high in nuts on lowering cholesterol levels. The beneficial effects of nut consumption observed in clinical and epidemiologic studies underscore the importance of distinguishing different types of fat. One study estimated that every exchange of one ounce of saturated fat to one once of nut-fat from consuming a whole nut was associated with a 45 percent reduction in heart disease risk.[2]

Study after study shows that raw nuts and seeds not only lower cholesterol, but also extend lifespan and protect against common diseases of aging. They also provide a good source of protein, which makes up about 15 to 25 percent of their calories.[3] Nuts' hard shells also keep them well protected from pesticides and environmental pollution. Raw nuts and seeds, not the salted or roasted variety, provide the most health benefits.

Over the last few years, the health benefits of seeds also have become more apparent. A tablespoon of ground flaxseed, hempseeds, chia seeds, or other seeds can supply those hard-to-find omega-3 fats that protect against diabetes, heart disease, and cancer.[4] Seeds are also rich in lignans, a type of fiber associated with a reduced risk of both breast cancer and prostate cancer. In addition, seeds are a good source of iron, zinc, calcium, protein, potassium, magnesium, Vitamin E, and folate. The plant goes to great effort in producing and protecting its seed, filling each genetic package with high concentrations of vitamins, minerals, proteins, essential oils, and enzymes.

While nuts and seeds have great health benefits, they are higher in calories and fat compared to vegetables, beans, and fruits so they should be consumed in smaller amounts. Nuts and seeds contain about 175 calories per ounce, and a handful could be a little over one ounce. For most of us, they are not a food that should be eaten in unlimited quantity. Unless you are thin and exercising frequently, hold your consumption of raw nuts and seeds to less than two ounces a day. In Book Two, I will demonstrate how these disease-fighting foods can be used to make delicious salad dressings and dips.

Eating Seeds and Nuts To Lose Weight

If you are significantly overweight and want to maximize your weight loss, you should limit your intake of seeds, nuts and avocados to one (one ounce) serving a day since they are calorie-rich. However, you should not exclude these healthy, high-fat foods completely from your diet. Although it may seem illogical to include such high fat foods in your diet (since fat is 9 calories a gram compared with 4 calories a gram for carbohydrates and protein), epidemiological studies show an inverse relationship between seed and nut consumption and body weight. Interestingly, these studies show including some seeds and nuts in your diet actually aids in appetite suppression and weight loss. Well-controlled trials that looked to see if eating nuts and seeds resulted in weight gain found the opposite; eating raw nuts and seeds promoted weight loss, not weight gain.[5] Because seeds and nuts are rich in minerals and fiber and have a low glycemic index, they are favorable foods to include in a diet designed for diabetics and even the obese. Researchers noted that people eating one ounce of nuts five times a week reduced their risk of developing diabetes by 27 percent.[6]

There is another important reason to include nuts and seeds in your diet as you lose weight and that is they prevent the formation of gallstones. Weight loss in general can increase one's risk of gallstone formation, but certainly that is a reasonable risk to take when one considers the ill-health and life-threatening effects from significant body fat. It is important to note, as reported in the American Journal of Clinical Nutrition, that when over 80,000 women were followed for 20 years it was found that the regular consumption of nuts and seeds offered dramatic protection against gallstone formation. These findings have also been duplicated in men.[7]

The health properties of nuts and seeds notwithstanding, it is important that you do not overeat them. Don't sit in front of the TV and eat an entire bag of nuts in an hour. Healthful eating means avoiding excessive calories and not eating for recreation. Besides being aware of the amount of seeds and nuts consumed, the only other modification that one needs to make to maximize weight loss in a plant-based diet is to limit the consumption of flour-containing baked goods and oils. Your carbohydrate consumption should come mostly from fresh fruit, squashes, carrots, peas and beans, not bread. And of course, your fat consumption should come from seeds and nuts, not oils.

Eating To Gain Weight

If you are slim or desirous of gaining weight, a larger amount of seeds, nuts and avocado is appropriate. The amount you should consume is based on your body weight, how much fat you have on your body, and how much you exercise. A pregnant or nursing woman should consume about two ounces of seeds and nuts a day, even if overweight, and may consume more than that if slim. A competitive athlete may require 4 – 6 ounces of raw seeds and nuts a day, in addition to an avocado. In other words, some of us have a higher requirement for these higher-protein, higher-fat foods, and others need less. We do not need as much fat in our diet when we have extra fat on our body that needs to be utilized for energy, but if we are thin (and especially if your physical activity level is high) we may have a substantially higher requirement for fat and calories. So even though we need to consume a significant amount of the lower calorie, very high micronutrient foods, some of these higher calorie foods are also important to fuel our caloric needs.

I provide nutritional counseling to world class and professional athletes to maximize their performance and to increase their resistance to infection. One key feature of the eating-style I recommend to them is that most of their protein and fat needs are met by consuming seeds, nuts, legumes and avocados instead of more animal products. I am not suggesting that these highly active individuals eat a low-fat diet. Rather, it is a diet with lots of healthy, whole-food fats from seeds, nuts and avocados. A diet with fifteen percent of calories from fat could be appropriate for an overweight person with heart disease, but a slim, healthy person may find 30 percent of calories from fat is more appropriate to their needs. A highly active teenager or athlete may function best on a diet that is 40 percent of calories from fat or more.

Most healthy, normal weight individuals who exercise moderately and are in good shape can eat 3 – 4 ounces of seeds and nuts a day. That will bring their fat intake up to about 30 percent of total calories. Believing fat is the villain is wrong. Eating a bread, potato, and pasta-based diet is not as healthful as a diet higher in fat, where the extra calories (and extra fat and protein) come from seeds and nuts. Eating more beans and whole grains can also be helpful for a person who wants to gain weight. Do not be tempted to eat more animal products to gain weight and don't get sucked in by the myth that you need more animal products to build muscle.

Keep in mind that eating to maintain extra fat stores on your body, because you or others think you look better heavier, is never healthful. A healthy person is slim and muscular. If you think you are too thin and desire more weight on your frame, the right way to achieve that is from working out in the gym, not in the kitchen. The muscular demands on your body will then increase your appetite, hunger will occur more frequently, and your caloric intake will increase proportionally to the increased muscular demand. If you want to gain weight, try to make your thighs, shoulders and chest a little bigger with more exercise. Don't expand your waistline by over-exercising your knife and fork.

CHAPTER ELEVEN

PHASE THREE IN PRACTICE

Thinking about Hunger in Your Life

Most Americans are overweight. This is to be expected. People should expect to become overweight when they do not meet their needs for nutrients and volume. It makes them into a food addict, and they are forced to overeat on calories. Processed foods, low-nutrient eating, and high-protein diets based on animal products create food addictions and derail true hunger.

Understanding and managing your hunger is a critical key to creating the physical environment that will deliver longevity and superior health. The body's drive to feed itself is part of the design to maintain optimal health and an ideal weight. It is geared toward self-preservation and its purpose is to make the body thrive. The irony is that people seem to have appetites bent on self-destruction. These are unnatural appetites. Our ability to enjoy unhealthy foods is the result of an otherwise useful ability to adapt to a variety of environments. This was useful in the past when food was scarce. Processed and unhealthy choices were unavailable. Our tastes were designed to enable us to enjoy whatever food we could obtain from the natural environment. It helped us to distinguish foods from poisons. In today's toxic food environment, the survival drive for calories could direct us to the most calorie-concentrated processed foods. Our innate drive for calories has been shackled by the food manufacturers peddling white flour, sweeteners, and artificial flavors. The more you eat low-nutrient, processed foods, the more those foods are craved. It is almost impossible not to over-consume calories and gain weight when your diet is so low in nutrients.

However, once you learn how to prefer the healthiest foods, managing your hunger boils down to structuring your eating so you consume the maximum nutrition in the fewest calories. If you consume adequate volume and nutrients, the calories will take care of themselves. The nerves lining the digestive tract send signals up to the brain, which control signals regulating eating behavior. When our nutrient and volume needs are unfulfilled, we desire more calories to feel satisfied, and we create food addictions.

When you eat with a focus on maximizing micronutrients in relation to calories, your body function will normalize, chronic illnesses like high blood pressure, diabetes, and high cholesterol will melt away, and you will maintain your youthful vigor into old age. You may be surprised to find that excess weight drops off at a relatively fast rate, without you even trying to diet or eat less. A consistent, ideal weight is easy to maintain when nutrient needs are met with an eating-style rich in vegetables, beans, and fresh fruits. You simply don't crave to overeat anymore. It's as if you had your stomach stapled, because once the micronutrient needs are met, it becomes difficult to overeat.

As you move into the Phase Three menus and recipes in Book Two, you will see the advice of this section turned into action in the supermarket and in the kitchen, where your choices determine your health destiny. As you are putting this knowledge into practice in your life, remember to take the time to think about what you're feeling before you start eating. If you think what you're experiencing is toxic hunger or an addiction, think if it is possible to delay eating a bit, or only eat something very healthy and light to stop the ill feeling. Don't worry. If you keep eating correctly and slowly stop overeating, these uncomfortable symptoms will slowly fade away.

As you eat healthier, high-nutrient foods and exclude unhealthier, low-nutrient foods in a manner that does not neglect the enjoyment of eating, you will find that your beliefs about what is possible will begin to change. You will see that eating healthfully really does not have to be a chore. You will be in control of your health and be able to make choices to live a long and disease-free life. You will see it is possible to slow the aging process. It is possible to prefer the healthiest foods. It is possible to miraculously transform your body.

Our lives are deterministically governed by the law of cause and effect. If we can adopt the right "cause," we will obtain the desired "effect."

I want you to write a description about yourself as the person you want to be two years from now, when you are in better health and have achieved all of your health goals. Visualize your body completely transformed by nutritional excellence with all the weight loss you want and the health attributes you want to earn. Use this to remind yourself of the person that you want to become.

ME TWO YEARS FROM NOW

TODAYS DATE _____

TWO YEARS FROM NOW DATE _____

WHO I WILL BE THEN:

_____

_____

_____

_____

Exercises with Food™
As you already know from practicing the Exercises with Food™ that you learned in Phases One and Two, these activities can help increase your pleasure derived from natural food and can help you adjust to eating with the goal of nutritional excellence. Like all exercises, they require frequent practice in order to see results.

Continue doing the previous Exercises with Food,™ with a particular focus on the palate stretching. This will help you rid yourself of toxic hunger. In addition, during this phase I want you to purposefully eat a light lunch or a light breakfast each day. Eating one lighter meal without snacking before the next meal, either lunch or dinner, will increase your true hunger before that meal. Over time, this will help to teach you what true hunger feels like. The main exercise target for this phase is to see if you can get back in touch with sensa-tions of "true hunger," differentiating the sensation from "toxic hunger." Be patient because it may take some time for toxic hunger to go away. It will help if you could link together an entire week of nutritional excellence so you can lose the toxic hunger symptoms and begin the pleasurable sensation of true hunger.

Phase Three Performance Goals
The menus and recipes in Book Two that correspond to Phase Three will take you to a new level of nutritional excellence. Try to reach these goals to further your journey.

- Continue the Exercises from Phases One and Two and supplement them with the new Exercise (above).

- Remove or greatly reduce red meat and cheese from your diet.

- Use the nut-based salad dressings found in Book Two, instead of oil-based ones.

- Eat high-vegetable dinners, with both raw greens and cooked greens and do not use animal products more than one serving every other day.

- Eliminate white flour and white sugar from your diet.

Clearly this is not an all or nothing plan. You will have fun, enjoy food, and eat for pleasure. However, it is important that mental obstacles don't prevent you from achieving your goals and protecting your health. Remember, no matter what phase and level of nutritional excellence you are on, you are navigating through life – making choices considering your health and your pleasure. We are all doing the same. As we learn and adapt to the heightened pleasures in life that are made available when you take excellent care of your health, we gain more pleasure from both our eating style and our life in general. Congratulations for seeking out the great pleasure available to you, simply through changing your diet, when you *Eat For Health*.

LIVING NUTRITIONAL EXCELLENCE

In this Phase of the program, you are studying and practicing at the pinnacle of nutritional excellence. In the next two chapters, you will learn more about the health impact of specific foods and how to take your diet to the most superior levels. This Phase will give you added tips, tricks, and techniques that will help you truly enjoy the healthiest eating-style on earth. For those of you who are willing to take it up a notch to strive for maximum health and longevity, Phase Four is for you. However, reaching and practicing Phase Four doesn't mean that you must be perfect in how you put it into practice every day of your life. It means that you have all the knowledge you need to maintain your commitment to nutritional excellence. It is here that you are giving your body the greatest opportunity to reach its ideal weight and the greatest chance of a full recovery if you have a chronic disease. If you are in good shape, you will gain the greatest chance to be free of diseases and to push the envelope of human longevity.

CHAPTER TWELVE

KEEPING FOCUS

"After three heart attacks within three months of each other and five angioplasties in a three-year period, I was still very ill. I almost died soon after the last angioplasty and had internal bleeding that was difficult to stop. The torture of all my medical problems made me think I would be better off if I had died. I was left with unstable angina, meaning I had chest pain from my bad heart almost constantly. I weighed 225 pounds and I could not walk one block. I was on ten medications and I was a cardiac cripple at the age of 60.

Luckily, I learned about Dr. Fuhrman and read his book, *Eat To Live*. Within three months of following the plan, my chest pain was gone, and I was walking again. From not being able to walk one block, I was able to walk two miles with no problems. Within seven months of eating Dr. Fuhrman's high-nutrient density plan, I weighed 135 pounds. I just wanted to be healthier and live again, but, in doing so, I had lost 90 pounds without even trying to lose weight.

When I think back to how sick I was, it is frightening. In addition to my other ailments, I suffered from daily migraines and had bleeding ulcers from all the medications I took. Now I walk three miles a day, go to yoga, exercise, and enjoy life immensely. I know I would not be alive today if not for Dr. Fuhrman's plan."

Julia Spano
Colonia, New Jersey

Health's Three Components

Congratulations! Whether you are just at the point of reading this section or you are actually ready to put Phase Four into practice in your life, getting here means you are motivated to make your health the best it can be. If you felt compelled to begin this journey, it was likely instinct that was driving you. Every living organism has a built-in thrive and survive instinct. Since you have been on the path towards maximizing your health for some time, you are likely now at the point where this type of nutrient-rich eating is beginning to become second nature. By being consistent in putting your newly obtained knowledge into practice, it is becoming ingrained as your healthy, new way of living. You are probably feeling a lot better than before, have lost a significant amount of weight if you needed to, and have the impetus to feel even better. In this Phase, I will be giving you additional information to further your path to great health.

Many people invest in their financial future but never consider their health future. The way you take care of yourself is just as crucial a determinant of your future happiness as your savings account. A large nest egg is of no use to you if you're not there to spend it! As you plan for your health future, you must consider the three important components that pay you back with high returns: your nutritional, physical, and social states. Each factor must be considered when the desire for the healthiest life possible is at stake.

- Nutritional Component Make every calorie count as you strive for maximum nutrition. Remember my health equation, $H = N/C$. Strive to eat high on the nutrient-density line.

- Physical Component Make physical exercise a part of your normal routine. Joining a gym is a great bonus, but learn to exploit all of the other opportunities in your life to exercise your body during the normal course of the day. Take the stairs instead of the elevator. Walk instead of riding when possible. Once you embrace nutritional excellence, you can strive for physical excellence. You may find that exercise becomes easier and more pleasurable with better health and a lower weight.

- Social Component Build a strong mental defense against unhealthy influences. A healthy mindset is a prerequisite for a healthy lifestyle, and the best way to develop it is to be optimistic and surround yourself with people who engage in and support your health. Even if you don't feel naturally optimistic, you can learn the attitude. Just reading this book shows you are optimistic. You know that you can earn great health and even create positive changes in your life!

The above three factors are all healthy habits that will eventually become second nature. The more you do them, the more they become your preferred way of life. Many unhealthy and healthy people are obsessed with food. Eating the right foods will make you incredibly healthy, but avoid obsessions even with healthy foods. They are often indicators of compulsions and other social issues. Striking a balance between eating and not eating is an excellent way to eliminate the obsession and strive for a fully balanced life where people, food, pleasure, recreation, exercise, work, rest, and sleep all have their place. The key to finding food's place in this balance is making the material you're learning instinctive and a natural part of an enjoyable life.

Addictions also make attempts at dietary modifications more difficult, but it only takes a few seconds of decision-making to win the battle and say an emphatic "no" to the addiction and "yes" to your new healthful lifestyle. I want to mention again that I have observed thousands of cases in which these positive changes have resulted in some temporary discomfort as the body eliminates toxins and restores its cells to a more youthful, decongested state. This is normal, and coping with it on the road to better health will be a small price to pay.

By now, some change has certainly occurred in your life as a result of learning this body of knowledge and applying the dietary guidelines and recipes found here. Do not underestimate the self-healing power of the human body once nutritional excellence is put into place and dietary and emotional stresses are removed. Many people have made these changes and have made complete recoveries from chronic illnesses that their doctors told them they would have forever.

During the vast majority of human history getting adequate calories was a difficult struggle. In those days, malnutrition from food scarcity was the major problem, not obesity. Humans are able to survive in so many environments because we are the most adaptable species on the planet, but our adaptability has become a liability because unhealthy options have become so accessible. However, you can control the choices that you make in that environment and strive to improve your health in all three components in your life. This book is about change and restoration. Hopefully, it will spur you to confront your fears about different dietary choices, reclaim your natural tastes, and restore your natural hunger drive.

The Stubborn Habits

So, you've learned which foods are best for your body, you've acquired some great recipes, and you are able to eat to your heart's content. All your problems are solved. Or are they? Do you still crave foods that you know are bad for you even when you aren't hungry? Let's talk briefly again about addiction and how to get beyond it.

Modern foods are designed to seduce your taste buds. You have been manipulated by profit-motivated food manufacturers. We all have. The artificially concentrated flavors that the processed food industry uses to stimulate the brain's pleasure center are designed to increase and retain sales. Tragically, the result is that they lead people's taste buds astray. Artificial, intense flavors cause us to enjoy natural flavors less. Our taste buds become desensitized, and the more we succumb to the heightened, artificial flavors, the less appealing natural, whole foods become. We discussed in Chapter Nine that salt also desensitizes our taste buds, but the extra sweeteners and artificial flavors combined with the flavor enhancing qualities of salt are all addictive.

Fortunately, by practicing this eating-style, your taste buds are bouncing back. However, it might take more time to reset your receptors to appreciate the more subtle flavors of whole, unprocessed foods. Hang in there, and keep up your healthy eating! It's the only way for this to happen, and it always does. It might take longer than six weeks, but your taste and flavor sensitivity will improve tremendously over time.

Realizing your impediments and gaining knowledge about great health are tremendous first steps, but they are only 50 percent of the overall solution. You must put into practice and repeat your new beneficial behaviors over and over until they become part of you. Repetition will make these positive actions feel more and more natural. It is not enough simply to know what to do. You need to practice preparing recipes, eating super-healthy meals, noticing the changes, and affirming yourself, until eating for health naturally satisfies you.

Developing a burning desire for optimal health will help you in the process of re-sensitizing your taste buds. Stay with the program and your taste buds will actually line up with your desire, your behaviors will line up with your beliefs, you will cease to crave flavor enhancers and highly seasoned food, and you will transform into a person who actually prefers to eat healthfully. As you learn more recipes, you will be able to substitute similar, healthy foods for those old, unhealthy options. For example, my healthy sorbets and ice creams are the perfect substitute for your craving of cold sweets.

It is not easy to develop new habits, and there is no such thing as a quick shortcut to developing new skills and expertise. When you do something over and over, it creates a pathway in the brain that makes it easier and more comfortable to repeat again. That is one reason why it is so hard to change bad habits. However, if you are motivated to persevere and keep trying, the change becomes considerably easier. The more you make healthful meals and the more days you link together eating healthful foods, the more your brain will naturally prefer to eat that way. Of course, feeling better and losing weight is a great motivator, but through this process, your taste for a different way of eating can be established. It has been shown that a new food needs to be eaten about 15 times for it to become a preferred food. Keep in mind that the more days you eat healthfully, the more you will lose your addiction to unhealthful, stimulating substances, and, with time, you will look forward to, and prefer, a healthy diet. Don't give up. The only failure is to stop trying.

Planning and Exercise

The ability to make the right decision consistently requires planning. You need time to prepare your environment so that you have good-tasting, healthy foods around you at all times to minimize temptation. Because eating healthfully has only gained popularity in recent years, few restaurants and quick food places make eating this way convenient. And because most of us work, it can be tough to fit everything, including cooking and exercise, into our busy schedules. Therefore, if you are going to succeed at turning your health or weight around, you will need to organize your time.

This book is not about exercise, but it is still important to mention that, without regular exercise, you cannot expect great health benefits. For excellent health in our later years, excellent nutrition must go hand in hand with regular, rigorous exercise. Our muscles and bones will shrink and weaken as we age if we do not exercise regularly and place demands on our skeleton. Osteoporosis is mostly the result of a sedentary lifestyle. If you shop and cook twice each week, you can still have time to exercise on the other days. Plenty of people exercise four times per week by following a schedule such as this: exercise once on Saturday, once on Sunday, and then two more times during the week. Below is a sample of a schedule of eating plans and exercising that you can modify for your own needs.

SAMPLE WEEKLY SCHEDULE		
Saturday	Eat out or take out food or salad bar	Exercise A
Sunday	Shop and cook today	Exercise B
Monday	Eat leftovers	
Tuesday	Eat leftovers	Exercise A
Wednesday	Shop and cook today	
Thursday	Eat leftovers	Exercise B
Friday	Eat leftovers	

Exercise A days, people typically walk uphill on an incline treadmill, skip rope, or ride a bike, and work out their abs, lower back and chest. Even 15 minutes of heart-beat-elevating, calorie-burning cardio, such as walking on a steep incline or pedaling on an elliptical machine, is good. If using a treadmill, gradually increase the incline as your cardiovascular fitness and exercise tolerance improves. Exercise B days, people typically exercise on an elliptical machine or a stair-climber and then work out legs, biceps, triceps, latissmus dorsi, and trapezius with weights or resistance. Aim for some cardio activities with an elevated pulse four times a week.

Make a list of all the exercises that you like to do and separate them into two different workouts. For example, make the A day easier on the thighs and B day heavier on the thighs so that you will be able to handle the B exercise day, even if it is the next day, without having your legs feel too tired.

Your exercise schedule and what exercises or activities you do should be individualized to your needs and preferences. The underlying theme is to plan it into your schedule. Do not exercise the same body parts in consecutive days, and spread out many different exercises to encompass various body parts into your weekly plan. If you are new to exercise, start slowly so you do not injure yourself. Begin by walking on a tread mill with only a three or four degree incline and lifting some very light dumbbells. Over time, keep increasing the incline on the treadmill, so you can eventually perform a more vigorous workout and burn more calories in your time allotment. Only increase speed on the treadmill after your increasing fitness level has enabled you to perform comfortably at the highest incline. It is better to go slower at a higher incline, than go faster at a lower incline. It puts less stress on your joints and you burn more calories. If you belong to a fitness facility or have access to a fitness professional, inquire about other exercises and the proper form of your workouts. Don't push yourself too hard, but make sure that you are doing physical exercise at least three times per week.

If you are significantly overweight, diabetic or have heart disease and your capacity for vigorous exercise is low, you will need to exercise more frequently, even two or three times a day. The lower your fitness level and the lower the intensity of exercise that you are capable of, the more frequently you need to exercise. Many of my patients with diabetes exercise twice daily. It is like their medicine before lunch and dinner. Even ten minutes of exercise, done regularly, is better than no exercise.

The better you plan out your weekly schedule in advance, the easier it will be to ingrain your new habits into your life. We live busy lives, we work hard, and we have to plan even our recreational activities and vacations in advance. So, make a weekly health plan and figure out:

- When you are going to shop

- What you are going to purchase when you shop.
  Be sure to make a list!

- What dishes, soups, or dressings you are going to
  prepare when you cook

- What dishes are made in large volume for use on
  multiple days and stored in the refrigerator or frozen

- What veggies and fruits you are going to have on
  hand frozen

- When you are going to exercise

- What exercises or activities you are going to do

- When you will go to sleep and wake up

- How relaxation, entertainment, and social activities
  can fit in and can be planned

Remember, not only does regular exercise burn calories during the time you are actually exercising, it also increases the caloric needs of your body into the days ahead, even on the days you are not exercising. It will work with your new eating-style to deliver dramatic benefits. **Exercise is the only way to increase your metabolic rate, healthfully.**

CHAPTER THIRTEEN

CLOSING IN ON GREAT HEALTH

Learn to Love Salads

Hundreds of population studies show that raw vegetable consumption offers strong protection against cancer.[1] The National Cancer Institute recently reported on over 300 different studies that all showed the same basic information: if consumed in large enough quantities, vegetables and fruits protect against all types of cancers, and raw vegetables have the most powerful anti-cancer properties of all foods.[2] However, less than one in 100 Americans consumes enough calories from raw vegetables to ensure this defense! I encourage my patients to eat two salads each day (or one salad and one green smoothie, which is discussed later in this chapter), and a glass of freshly squeezed vegetable juice whenever possible. To help you remember the importance of raw vegetables, put a big sign on your refrigerator that says, **"The Salad is the Main Dish."**

The word salad here means any vegetable eaten raw or uncooked. Fresh fruit, unsulfured dried fruits, canned beans, and a delicious dressing can be added to it. **Eating a huge, delicious salad is the secret to successful weight control and a long healthy life.**

This health makeover program encourages you to eat raw vegetables in unlimited quantities, but think big. Since they have a negative caloric effect, the more you eat, the more weight you will lose. Raw foods also have a faster transit time through the digestive tract, resulting in more weight loss than their cooked counterparts. The objective is to eat as many raw vegetables as possible, with the goal of one-pound daily. An easy way to accomplish this is to eat a salad at the beginning of your lunch, and then have some raw vegetables with dip before dinner. This could be an entire head of lettuce with one or two tomatoes and some shredded peppers, beets, or carrots. Or, you could have cucumber and shredded cabbage with shredded apples and raisins, or raw broccoli, cherry tomatoes, and snow pea pods with a delicious humus or salsa dip. The possibilities are endless, and Book Two details many ways for you to reach this goal. Though it may seem daunting, it is far from impossible to consume one pound of raw vegetables, especially if it is split between two meals. Believe it or not, an entire pound is less than 100 calories of food.

My long-time advice to eat a large amount of raw vegetables—a.k.a. a salad—before lunch and dinner has been tested by the medical community. Researchers used a crossover design to track the calories consumed by the same people when they ate salads as an additional first course at a meal and when they didn't. The research showed that consuming salads reduces meal-calorie intake and is an effective strategy for weight control.[3] Raw vegetables are not only for weight control; they also promote superior health in general.

When you add one of my delicious fruit, nut, or avocado-based dressings to the salad, the monounsaturated fats in the dressing increase the body's ability to absorb the anti-cancer compounds in the raw vegetables.[4] The synergistic combination of the raw vegetables and the healthy dressing makes the salad a health food superhero.

Greens Are King

As we've discussed, all foods get their calories from fat, carbohydrate, or protein. Green vegetables, unlike high-starch vegetables like carrots and potatoes, get the majority of their calories from protein. When more of your protein needs are met from green vegetables, you get the benefit of ingesting a huge amount of critical, life-extending micronutrients.

The biggest animals all eat predominantly green vegetation, gaining their size from the protein found there. Obviously, greens pack a powerful, nutrient-dense punch. Some high-green-eating animals—primates—have a very similar biology and physiology to humans. Based on genetic information, chimpanzee and human DNA only differs by 1.6 percent. The desire of primates for variety in their diet supports nutrient diversity that enables them to live a long life, free of chronic diseases. But, without an adequate amount of plant-derived nutrients, immune system dysfunction develops. The results of a compromised immune system are frequent infections, allergies, autoimmune disease, and often cancer. The micronutrients that fuel the primate immune system are found in nature's cupboard—the garden and forest.

Now that you have delved this far into the field of nutritional medicine, you might as well invest a few more health dollars in your body's nutrient bank account by focusing on your consumption of greens every day. Low in calories and high in life-extending nutrients, green foods are your secret weapon to achieve incredible health. Scientific research has shown a strong positive association between the consumption of green vegetables and a reduction of all the leading causes of death in humans.[5] Cruciferous vegetables—in particular broccoli, Brussels sprouts, cabbage, kale, bok choy, collards, watercress, and arugula, to name a few—are loaded with disease-protecting micronutrients and powerful compounds that promote detoxification.

To bring your body to a phenomenal level of health, my aim is to deliver these foods to your plate in a variety of ways that make them delicious and increase your absorption of their beneficial nutrients. Greens can be served raw in salads, steamed and chopped as part of dinner, and cooked in soups. When we steam or boil vegetables some of the phytochemicals, vitamins, and minerals get lost in the water, but when we simmer vegetables in soup, all the nutrients are retained in the liquid. Additionally, the liquid base of the soup prevents the formation of toxic compounds that are created as food is browned under dry heat. Many beneficial chemical compounds are more readily absorbed when the food has been softened with heat.[6] If you have been studying the recipes and menus in Book Two, you have found that we incorporate larger quantities of greens in an assortment of delicious ways as you move up the stages of dietary excellence.

Juicing and Blending

All plants are composed of cells whose walls consist mainly of cellulose, a type of carbohydrate. Humans do not have the enzyme capable of breaking down cellulose, so we cannot utilize cellulose as an energy source. The only way we can break down these walls and release the most nutrients possible from the cells into the bloodstream is by thoroughly chewing fruits and vegetables. However, when we chew a salad, we often don't do an efficient job of crushing every cell; about 70 to 90 percent of the cells are not broken open. As a result, most of the valuable nutrients contained within those cells never enter our bloodstream and are lost. They just travel through our bodies until they are excreted. This is one of the reasons why practicing the chewing exercises detailed in Phase One is so important to the *Eat For Health* plan.

An even more efficient way to ensure you receive these needed nutrients is using a blender to puree raw, leafy greens. The blending process aids your body in the work of breaking down and assimilating nutrients. It guarantees that a higher percentage of nutrients will be absorbed into your bloodstream. If you add a glass of freshly squeezed vegetable juice to your diet periodically or daily, you can pump up your vegetable consumption easily and increase the availability and absorption of the anti-cancer phytochemical compounds.

Making green smoothies or *blended salads* is also a delicious and convenient way to pump up your consumption of greens. It is amazing how many people love the taste of these liquefied mixtures of raw greens and fruit that can be made in a high-powered blender. While you sip or eat a creamy smooth blended salad with a spoon, think about all of the nutrients that are now powering your body to restore and maintain optimal health. Savory blended salads can be made with endless combinations of vegetables, nuts, herbs, and condiments. They can be made to taste like gazpacho, creamy summer soups, a fruit shake, or a salad dressing. My typical green smoothie blends two ounces of lettuce, two ounces of spinach, a banana, a date, and half an avocado. You will find several delicious green smoothie (blended salad) recipes in Book Two.

If you have a digestive disorder, blending and juicing vegetables can be a great aid because you can increase your consumption of healing nutrients, even though your digestive capacity might be sub-par. Since eating a low-phyto-chemical, low-fiber diet goes against nature's design and causes most digestive disorders, eating a high-nutrient, vegetable-based diet often resolves digestive problems quickly. People suffering from irritable bowel syndrome, constipation, hemorrhoids, and reflux disease often see improvements after just a few weeks of juicing and eating blended salads. However, sometimes diets have to be modified for individual uniqueness or medical problems, such as ulcerative colitis or Crohn's disease, conditions that require fresh fruits and raw vegetables to be gradually introduced into the diet. In such cases, working with a knowledgeable physician may be helpful.

The high-nutrient availability of blended vegetables also helps normalize immune function in those suffering from asthma, allergies, and other immune system disorders. High-performance athletes or those interested in gaining weight can mix nuts and seeds into their blended vegetables. This combination supplies healthy sources of protein and fat in an efficiently absorbed, high-nutrient package.

Fresh Fruits Fight Cancer

Fresh fruits are an important component of the natural diet of all primates. Humans and other primates have color vision and the ability to appreciate sweets. We are designed this way so that we can recognize ripe fruits and be attracted to them. We have a natural sweet tooth designed to direct us to those foods most critical for our survival, but sugar and candy manufacturers also know that bright colors and sweet tastes are instinctually attractive. They have used that knowledge to their advantage. Remember, your instinctual reaction is designed to lead you to fruit—not sugary, processed foods. Fruit is an indispensable requirement to maintain a high level of health. Fruit consumption has been shown to offer the strongest protection against certain cancers, especially oral, esophageal, lung, prostate, and pancreatic cancer.[7]

Researchers also have discovered substances in fruit that have unique effects on preventing aging and deterioration of the brain. Some fruits, particularly berries, are rich in phytochemicals that have anti-aging effects. Berries are an excellent, nutrient-dense, low-calorie source of vitamins and phytochemicals. Researchers have seen that blueberries also have protective effects for brain health in later life.[8] In addition, certain pectins—natural parts of the cellular makeup of fruits such as oranges, kiwis, and pomegranates—also lower cholesterol and protect against cardiovascular disease.[9]

As you can see, fruit is vital to your health and well-being and can contribute to lengthening your life. While our natural, sweet desires are usually satisfied by convenient treats, we can use fresh and frozen fruits to make delicious desserts that are healthy and taste great. Book Two provides many delicious and easy fruit recipes to satisfy your sweet tooth in a healthy manner. When you complete your evening meal with one of those recipes—a frozen strawberry sorbet, a cantaloupe slush, or simply a bowl of fresh berries—you are putting the finishing touches on a meal that will satisfy your desire for a sweet food, while intellectually satisfying your desire to be healthy and wise.

Cut Back on Grains
As you well know by now, to eat healthfully, fruits and vegetables should form the base of your food pyramid. That means that grains should be consumed in a much smaller amount than you were most likely eating before you began this plan. Grains simply do not contain enough nutrients per calorie to form a substantial part of your diet.

SELECTED NUTRIENTS IN BREAD - POTATO - CORN - PEAS

	WHITE BREAD	WHOLE WHEAT	WHITE POTATO	CORN	PEAS
Potassium	37 mg	112 mg	575	232	323
Beta-Carotene	0	0.2	6.5	62	560
Lutein	16	32	32	898	3087
Magnesium	8.6	29	30	30	46
Folate	5	23	30	43	75
Vitamin C	0	0	10	5.3	17
Fiber	1	2.2	2.4	2.6	6.5

Many scientific studies show a strong association between the consumption of white flour products, such as pasta and bread, with diabetes, obesity, and heart disease.[10] Refined carbohydrates are also linked to enlargement of the prostate.[11] These results continue to show that eating white flour and sweeteners is nutritional suicide that will undermine your health.

Whole grains are the least nutrient-dense food of the seed family, and they do not show the powerful protection against disease that is apparent in the scientific studies of fresh fruit, vegetables, beans, raw nuts, or seeds. Just because a food is called whole grain or organic does not make it a good food. Many whole-grain cold cereals are so processed and overly cooked that they have lost most of their nutritional value. As was mentioned in Chapter Nine, because these foods were dry-baked to make them crisp, they are also generally high in acrylamides and other toxic compounds. Soaking, sprouting, or cooking grains in water, instead of eating pre-cooked breakfast cereals, is a much healthier and more nutritious way to eat them. Some of the healthier grains to consume include barley, buckwheat (kasha), millet, oats, quinoa, and wild rice. As a minor part of your diet, they can be water-cooked and used as a breakfast cereal with fruits and nuts or a dinner side dish.

White potato is also not a high-nutrient food, and many studies reveal an association between a diet high in white potato and obesity and diabetes.[12] Granted these studies may be biased by the way potatoes are consumed, often fried or loaded with butter or sour cream, but, nevertheless, because of their relatively low-nutrient density and their high glycemic index they should play a minor role in your diet. Sweet potatoes, carrots, and peas are much healthier options.

Fish Is Not a Health Food
Many people believe they are improving their diets by eating less meat and more fish. Since fish is generally low in fat and high in beneficial omega-3 fats, many consider it an important part of a healthy diet. Studies have demonstrated that when people eat less red meat and more fish, health outcomes are improved.

However, a review of the literature on fish consumption shows that fish is a double-edged sword because it is one of the most polluted foods we eat. In spite of the presence of valuable omega-3 fats, called EPA and DHA, nearly all fish and shellfish contain mercury and other pollutants, such as PCB's. Pollutants and mercury accumulate in fish as the polluted water is filtered through their gills. Larger fish that have lived longer have the highest levels of mercury because they've had more time to accumulate it. They may also accumulate it from all the smaller fish they have eaten, similar to the way we accumulate mercury in our tissues from the fish we eat. People who would be disgusted at the thought of drinking polluted water don't think twice about eating polluted fish that contain literally 100-times more pollution. As the below chart shows, no fish is free of pollution.

MERCURY AND OTHER POLLUTANTS IN VARIOUS SEAFOOD Source: FDA Surveys, 1990–2003	
HIGH MERCURY SEAFOOD	HIGH IN PCBs AND NON-MERCURY POLLUTANTS
King Mackerel Shark Whale Swordfish Tilefish Grouper Sea Bass Marlin Halibut Lobster Scorpion Fish Snapper	Salmon Sardines Herring Bluefish Lobster Catfish Clams and Oysters Crab

INTERMEDIATE MERCURY SEAFOOD	LOW MERCURY SEAFOOD
Tuna	Shrimp
Pike	Tilapia
Largemouth Bass	Haddock
Bluefish	Flounder
Carp	Scallops
Mahi Mahi	Squid
Mackerel (Gulf)	Trout
Monkfish	Hake
Orange Roughy	Ocean Perch
Cod	
Croaker	
Pollock	
Whitefish	
Sea Trout (Weakfish)	

If you eat fish regularly, your body is undoubtedly high in mercury. You cannot remove the mercury by trimming the fat or by cooking because it is deposited throughout the fish's tissues. Mercury levels tested in patients correlate exceptionally well with the amount of fish the individuals consumed. Individuals eating fish a few times a week had blood mercury levels exceeding 5.0 micrograms, the maximum level recommended by the National Academy of Sciences. Women eating seafood more than twice per week had seven times the blood mercury levels of non-fish eaters, and children eating fish regularly had mercury levels 40 times higher than the national mean.[13,14] Mercury can be removed from the body naturally, but, even after a patient avoids fish for a period of time, it may take years for the levels to drop significantly.

Though the FDA reassures us that we will not be harmed by acute mercury poisoning if we eat a variety of fish with different amounts of mercury, they do not guarantee we won't suffer from the continual accumulation of mercury over the years. As the recognition that mercury damages the brains of our children has increased in the last two decades, the EPA has lowered its recommendations for what it considers an acceptable level of mercury for pregnant women more than once. Over 300,000 newborns every year are thought to develop adverse neurodevelopmental effects of mercury exposure in utero. If something can damage a fetus and result in childhood learning abnormalities, it can't be considered something to promote as healthy for adults. If it's damaging cells in the fetus, you can bet adult cells are damaged too; we just may not see the damage in the short run. Along with other negative influences, subtle cellular damage from mercury can be a contributory factor that leads to the development of diseases later in life. High body stores of mercury cause brain damage and memory impairment, leading to dementia in later life, and the risks of such developments increase with age. High mercury levels can also cause hypertension, heart disease, mental disorders, and endocrine diseases.[15]

EPA and DHA fat in fish can have some blood-thinning effects to counter the inflammation caused by a high intake of animal products and saturated fat. Unfortunately, while fish oil has an anti-clotting effect like aspirin, the mercury in fish has the opposite effect and increases the risk of a heart attack. This is because mercury is cardio-toxic. Given this, the potential benefit of a fish's ability to thin the blood and counter the clot-promoting effects of a diet heavy in animal products is offset by the higher exposure to mercury. Multiple studies have shown that high intake of fish actually increases one's risk of coronary death.[16]

Fish consumption has also been found to have a dose-dependent relationship with breast cancer. Consumption of all types of fish—wild or farm raised; high or low in omega-3 fats—is linked to higher breast cancer rates. A Diet Cancer and Health study concluded, "Higher intake of fish was significantly associated with higher incidence rates of breast cancer."[17] Surprisingly, women consuming little or no fish were found to have approximately half the incidence of breast cancer compared to high fish consumers.[18]

If the consumption of toxins gleaned from fish has potential health risks, wouldn't it be better to get our omega-3 fats from a cleaner source? Yes. It is safer to rely on a clean, low-dose, DHA supplement, such as my DHA Purity, or a clean fish-oil supplement taken a few times a week instead of eating potentially dirty fish. Since my DHA Purity supplement is not fish-derived, you are assured of achieving adequate DHA levels without mercury and other pollutants. When buying these omega-3 supplements, keep in mind that they should be purchased from a well-documented, reliably clean source, close to the date of manufacturing, and refrigerated upon receipt.

The bottom line on fish is we can no longer consider it a health food. Either avoid it or eat it no more than once weekly. If you do have fish, chose from the lower-fat, lowest mercury types, such as tilapia, flounder, scallops, trout, or sole. Be aware of the place where it was caught and what type of fish it is. Never accept recreational fish from questionable waters, and never eat high-mercury-content fish. It is not worth the risk.

Phase Four in Practice

As you now know from reading about and practicing this eating-style, the most effective way to properly care for your health is to strive for nutritional excellence. To do that, you must stay focused on the nutrient quality of the food you eat. However, I want to reiterate, reaching this stage of the program doesn't demand perfection; nor does it mean that you will never eat meat again or that you will never have a slice of birthday cake. It means that your diet has been revamped so that high-nutrient fruits, vegetables, beans, and other foods make up the large majority of your food intake, and that you have the knowledge and skills to come even closer to nutritional excellence each day. The instances that you eat meat and cakes will be fewer, but you will undoubtedly find that, with time, those foods are less enjoyable. You may eventually choose not to eat them or other unhealthy foods because you have lost your desire and taste for them. As you strive to make your eating-style the healthiest it can be, remember the tips and techniques in this phase that can give you an extra boost towards that goal.

- Eliminate or reduce your consumption of fish to no more than once per week.

- Engage in physical activity four times per week.

- Make a diet, shopping, and exercise plan at the beginning of each week.

- Eat a blended salad or vegetable juice at least three times per week.

- Continue eating according to the nutritional guidelines in Book Two.

I hope that what you have read in this phase and in the rest of this book has shown you that there is a whole body of nutritional information that has never been shared with the general public. Even when health professionals are educated, the power of lifestyle intervention and dietary modifications to help people suffering with serious medical problems is hardly addressed because the emphasis is on intervention with pills, drugs, and surgeries. Commercial interests have dominated the nutritional message we have learned to date, and the medical profession has become infatuated with technological advancements. This approach has not only failed to improve the general health of our nation, but it has also resulted in a dramatic explosion of the diseases of nutritional ignorance and pushed health care spending through the roof without any improvement in healthy life expectancy to show for it.

I hope every one of you reading this book can use your life to prove the strength of nutrition by achieving enhanced vigor and great health and from your example encourage others to discover how rewarding it is to eat for health. Protecting yourself from a needless health tragedy is not only in your best interest, but is a gratifying experience that can bring satisfaction and pleasure to your life. Your success will encourage others to get healthy too. The power of *Eat For Health* is knowledge that we all deserve so that we can make critical choices for our own lives and take back control of our health.

CHAPTER FOURTEEN

FREQUENTLY ASKED QUESTIONS

Nutrition Confusion

"EAT ALL THE MEAT YOU LIKE."
"NEVER EAT MEAT."

"EAT MANY SMALL MEALS A DAY."
"EAT ONLY THREE MEALS A DAY."

"SOY IS BAD FOR YOU."
"SOY IS NECESSARY IN A HEALTHY DIET."

The list of contradictory advice about what constitutes a healthy diet goes on and on. With so much confusion and so many unverified claims floating around, it's understandable that many people give up on nutrition before they even get started. However, in having reached this point in this book, you have the knowledge to be unaffected by such statements. You now know that correct nutrition is founded on solid science and math. The truth is simple: for both optimal health and weight loss, you must consume a diet with a high nutrient-per-calorie ratio. Avoiding deficiencies and getting a full symphony of food-derived phytochemicals and antioxidants are the critical elements in creating a long, healthy life, free of the many diseases that are so common in America.

Many people don't have this knowledge, and they jump from one popular diet to another, or try one fad diet and then settle with less than optimal results.

Because popular diets are seldom backed by valid scientific evidence and rarely focus on nutritional excellence, they are doomed to fail. It is unlikely that traditional dieting will ever result in a slim and healthy body, unless you have changed your food preferences from unhealthy to healthy foods and rid your body of its addictions. Losing some weight and then gaining it back again is of no benefit. Only weight loss that you maintain forever offers long-term health improvement, which means diet changes only have real benefits if they become part of your permanent, everyday lifestyle, not something that you practice for a few months and then abandon. Making permanent changes can only come from being knowledgeable, seeing impressive results as a result of the application of that knowledge, and experiencing personal growth that sees these critical lifestyle changes as worthwhile and pleasurable.

In having come this far in *Eat For Health*, you have the knowledge that you need to make these permanent changes, but, since much of this information is contrary to what you have learned about food from other sources, you may still be experiencing some uncertainty. The questions and answers that follow are intended to help solidify and reinforce what you have learned so far and help clear up any confusion that may remain.

---

1. Isn't being overweight genetic? Can *Eat For Health* help those who have an overweight or obese family?

As we discussed in Chapter Six, the role that genetics plays in obesity is undeniable. People whose parents are obese have a ten-fold increased risk of becoming obese themselves. But the fraction of the population considered obese had doubled in the last 25 years, so, clearly, obesity is not primarily genetic. This is a new problem in human history that is the result of modern eating habits. Think about this: obese families tend to have obese pets. That kind of obesity is obviously not genetic. How humans and pets eat is different, but this anecdote helps to show that behavior and environment play a role in being overweight among those with a genetic predisposition. So, it is the combination of food choices, inactivity, and genetics that determines obesity.[1] Those who genetically store fat more efficiently may have had a survival advantage thousands of years ago when food was scarce, but in today's modern food pantry, where high-calorie, toxic foods abound, those people are at a survival disadvantage. Focusing on the element of genetics in the formula that adds up to obesity doesn't solve the problem. You can't change your genes. Rather than taking an honest look at what causes obesity, Americans are still looking for a magical, effortless cure for it—a gimmick, drug, or surgery. The only answer that is out there is living a healthy lifestyle focused on excellent nutrition along with adequate activity and exercise. If you live this way, the benefits will overwhelm genetics and allow even those with a genetic hindrance to weight loss to achieve a healthy weight.

One of the most exciting studies in the field of weight control and obesity in recent years was published in the New England Journal of Medicine.[2] This study documented that if you have a friend who is obese, your risk of developing obesity increases by close to 60 percent, a higher rate than if a sibling or even a spouse becomes obese. This high percentage held up even after controlling for the fact that people tend to form bonds with others similar to them. If both people listed each other as friends, and one became obese first, the second was approximately three times as likely to follow suit.

This illustrates that obesity is spread by similar eating styles in social networks. Peer influence is not to be underestimated. However, understanding how powerful bad influences can be, especially with society's approval and promotion of addictive eating, leads to the inescapable conclusion that healthful behaviors can be just as contagious if you are surrounded by health-conscious people. One powerful secret to a slim body and good health is to cultivate friends who are supportive and can share a healthy eating-style with you. Genetics are not the major factor. The social norms of the modern world have made obesity pervasive.

2. Aren't some conditions like heart disease and dementia inevitable as we age?

As this chart shows, heart disease as a major cause of disability and death is a recent phenomenon.

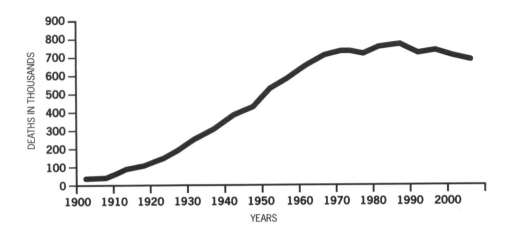

Heart disease was not inevitable in the past and it doesn't have to be inevitable now. It has known causes. Populations where these predisposing lifestyles are not lived out have practically no heart disease. When studies look at these issues, they find that the cultures that eat a healthy, vegetable-rich diet have almost no recorded heart disease, including hundreds of thousands of rural Chinese who have not had a single documented heart attack.[3] Because heart disease has become so ubiquitous in America, many people believe the myth that heart disease, high blood pressure, strokes, and dementia are largely genetic or the consequence of aging. It may be rare in the modern world that any majority of a population exercises, does not smoke, and eats very healthfully, but those that do earn a low-risk status and do not have heart attacks.[4]

The same factors that cause atherosclerosis, leading to heart attacks and strokes, also create dementia, and I am referring to both vascular dementia and Alzheimer's. This includes the same diets that are high in animal fat and low in vitamins, minerals, fruits, and green vegetables.[5] Of course, smoking and lack of physical exercise play a role in these common diseases, but the point is that it does not have to happen to you. These diseases, and others that plague modern America, are not the inevitable consequences of aging. They can actually resolve and improve with age or can be avoided entirely. They are simply the result of years of poor nutrition and an unhealthy lifestyle. My hope for you is that through this eating style, you, like my patients who have embraced this program, can rid yourself of migraine headaches, acne, autoimmune diseases, and diabetes. Many of my patients have restored their health after conventional physicians—and the conventional beliefs about the inevitability of disease— told them their problems were going to be life long. Their doctors were wrong.

3. **Through the four phases in this book, you have been reducing the intake of animal products until they are only consumed two or three times per week. Would a total vegetarian (vegan) diet be better for one's long-term health than one that includes these few servings?**

There is no clear scientific data that indicates a total vegetarian or vegan diet would be more lifespan-promoting than one with two or three servings of animal products per week. However, a high-nutrient, vegan diet-style can still be a healthy choice. The available research on the issue shows there is no clear answer, but a large amount of evidence supports the idea that there is not a large difference among diets that get zero to 15 percent of their calories from animal products, as long as the diet is otherwise micronutrient-rich. To play it safe and to maximize intake of plant-based nutrients, I recommend following this nutritarian plan and holding animal products to under ten percent of total calories. A diet that falls within this range is healthy and can maximize your health and lifespan. Following the recipes and meal plans in *Eat For Health* will allow you to easily live and eat in this range. However, if a person has heart disease, I would advise they adopt the strictest version of this plan either, vegan or with just one serving of fish per week, for maximal reversal of atherosclerosis.

Keep in mind that the overwhelming majority of Americans consume more than 40 percent of their calories from animal products, and some popular, high-protein diets recommend an even higher intake. The world's scientific literature is clear that for maximum health and longevity, this amount of animal product consumption must be dropped significantly.

A careful review of the science leads to the inescapable conclusion that animal products must be limited; the exact degree of that limitation is still up for debate. In my years of practice, I have infrequently encountered some individuals who had higher protein needs than could be easily met with a vegan diet. This finding was initiated with some complaint thought to be linked to their vegan diet and then confirmed with blood work showing low amino acid levels. When the diet was adjusted to put back a small amount of animal products or protein supplementation the difficulty often resolved. My first step in advising appropriate dietary modifications for these people was to include more plant proteins such as sunflower seeds and soybeans and whole food sources of fat, so if animal products are still indicated the amount needed would be minimal. Even these rare individuals, who showed a need for some animal-based foods in their diet, thrived with limiting animal product intake to three small servings per week.

Overall, for all people, varying animal intake between zero and three servings per week is likely to be healthful as long as the other elements of the diet are properly executed.

The longest lived population, living in the United States, is the Californian Seventh Day Adventists. When about 34,000 of them were followed between 1976 and 1988 it became apparent that those who adopted the Adventist-recommended healthy behaviors, which include veganism, flexitarian or near-vegan diets, lived about ten years longer than other Californians.[6] A review of 6 prospective cohort studies on long-term vegetarians and low meat intake from the Adventist Health Study confirmed that a very low meat intake was associated with significant increases in longevity.[7] This data was also corroborated in the massive China-Oxford-Cornell Study. For example, disease rates, for heart disease and cancer, continued to drop as people went from an average of seven servings of animal products per week to 1.7 servings per week.[8] A total vegan population was not studied in the China Study.

Of course a vegan diet requires a B12 supplement. Vitamin B12 is only found in foods of animal origin. If a vegan population was studied in the China Study, B12 deficiency would likely become an issue, weakening the advantage from a further drop in animal products. A primitive population eating a mostly vegetarian diet would still get enough B12 from some insect and bacterial contamination, but, today, a person following a completely vegan lifestyle needs to add a B12 vitamin supplement.

The other interesting and important observation on diet and longevity is that the longest lived populations (mentioned earlier) in the world such as Hunza in Central Asia, Vilcabamba in South America and Okinawa in Japan all show that these ultra-long-lived people eat a diet that is nutrient-rich, with 80 to 95 percent of calories coming from unrefined plant foods.[9] A diet rich in vegetables and very low in animal products is the hallmark of these ultra-long-lived societies.

Overall, epidemiologic studies point to the fact that the intake of unrefined plant food must be very high to assure very low rates of cancer and promote maximum lifespan in humans. The advantages gained from a vegetarian diet, particularly for disease reduction, are also because individuals not eating animal products are more likely consuming a greater amount of high-nutrient plant foods. The interaction between nutrient-rich plant food and the low intake of animal products is the key combination for dramatic advances in healthy life expectancy. So the critical issue for disease reduction is not whether one is a pure vegan or not; the issue is the micronutrient quality of the diet in conjunction with a comparatively low intake of animal products. In essence, one must be a nutritarian, which means you are a health-conscious eater whose primary dietary concern is to maximize nutrient density. The bottom line is that to live in the most health-promoting way, you must eat plenty of vegetables, fruits, and beans with some seeds and nuts, but you do not have to exclude all animal products.

4. **How do I get enough protein if I am only eating a few servings of animal products a week or less? Does your eating-style provide enough protein for athletes?**

Many people are still tied to the myth that a person needs to eat animal products every day or at every meal for his or her diet to be nutritionally sound. To add to the confusion is the myth that more protein will help you lose weight and more carbohydrates will inhibit weight loss. There is also a myth that vegetables must be combined within a meal to create amino acid patterns resembling those in animal foods in order to receive an adequate balance of protein.

Studies have shown that children and adults grow healthy and strong on vegetarian diets. While some vegetables have higher or lower proportions of certain amino acids than others, when eaten in amounts to satisfy an individual's caloric needs, a sufficient amount of all essential amino acids is provided.

Protein is ubiquitous. It is contained in all foods, not only animal products. Even if you ate nothing but plant foods, as long as your caloric requirements were met from wholesome, natural foods, you would have sufficient protein. Foods such as peas, green vegetables, and beans have more protein per calorie than meat. In addition, foods that are rich in plant protein are generally the foods that are richest in nutrients and phytochemicals. By eating more of these high-nutrient, low-calorie foods, we get plenty of protein, and our bodies get flooded with protective micronutrients simultaneously. Animal protein does not contain antioxidants and phytochemicals; plant protein does. Eating less animal protein and more plant protein is good for your heart and blood vessels. When you drop body fat, your cholesterol lowers somewhat, but when you reduce animal-protein intake and increase plant-protein intake, you lower cholesterol radically. Vegetables contain sufficient protein, have no saturated fat or cholesterol, and are higher in nutrients than any other food.

PROTEIN CONTENT FROM SELECTED PLANT FOOD

FOOD	GRAMS PROTEIN
Banana	1.2
Corn (one cup)	2
Brown rice (one cup)	5
Whole wheat bread (2 slices)	5
Spinach-frozen (one cup)	7
Peas-frozen (one cup)	9
Almonds 3 oz	10
Broccoli (two cups)	10
Tofu (4 ounces)	11
Sesame Seeds (1/2 cup)	12
Sunflower seeds (1/2 cup)	13
Kidney beans (one cup)	13
Chick Peas (one cup)	15
Lentils (one cup)	18
Soybeans (one cup)	29

Protein requirement studies of the 1950s demonstrated that adults require a minimum of 30 grams of protein per day.[10] Today, the average American consumes 100 to 120 grams of protein daily, mostly in the form of animal products. People who eat a plant-based diet have been found to consume 60 to 80 grams of protein each day, well above the minimum requirement.[11] The problem is the emphasis on trying to get more of something we are already getting too much of in our bodies. Protein deficiency in this country is extremely rare, except for people who are experiencing malabsorption due to illness. It is very unlikely that you need more protein unless you are eating an unbalanced diet that is deficient in many other ways as well.

Trying to eat more protein is just as disease-causing as trying to eat more carbohydrates or more fat. All of them are good if we are chronically malnourished, like a patient with anorexia, but they are all bad if we are already getting too much. If any exceeds our basic requirements, the excess hurts us. The excess protein you do not use is converted to fat or eliminated through the kidneys, accompanied by calcium and other minerals that are drawn from your bones, which can lead to osteoporosis and kidney stones.

It is true that resistance training and endurance workouts increase your need for protein, but it is proportional to the calories burned with the exercise. If you meet the increased demand for calories from a heavy workout with a healthy assortment of natural plant foods you will get the extra protein you need. You do not need to supplement with protein drinks and powders. Being physically fit is great, but eating to promote unnatural largeness is not lifespan-favorable. You may not be able to promote enough growth to become a linebacker, but who said size is equated with good health? Large athletes who have overeaten on animal products throughout their lives have six times the risk of early life death compared to less-muscled athletes.[12] Being that large is dangerous to your long-term health, even if it is not all fat.

Nevertheless, you can still get strong and muscular eating plant proteins. Even an enthusiastic body builder who wants to build one-half pound of extra muscle per week only needs approximately seven extra grams of protein per day. Exercise drives increased hunger, and, as the athlete consumes more calories to meet the demands of exercise, he or she will naturally get the extra protein they need. Consider my friend Ken

Williams, a world-class body builder who eats a vegan diet. He plans his diet to get sufficient protein. He needs more calories than you or I do because he exercises so much, so he eats more food, and he meets his increased protein needs.

Don't forget, the goal of a healthy diet is to get the most micronutrients per calorie, both in terms of amount and diversity. It is important not to consume excess calories. The focus on the importance of protein in a diet is one of the major reasons we have been led down the path to dietary suicide. We have equated protein with good nutrition while ignoring micronutrient content. Because of this, we have neglected vegetables, beans, nuts, and seeds, and have instead relied on animal products, believing they are the most favorable source of protein. We bought a false bill of goods, and the dairy and meat-heavy diets that have resulted created a tragic heart attack and cancer epidemic. So you do not have to worry about getting enough protein. Even a vegan version of the *Eat For Health* eating style, which focuses on high-nutrient plant sources of protein, gives you plenty of protein and it would be unusual for a person to require more.

5. How can I protect my bones? Don't I need an adequate amount of dairy and milk for calcium and to prevent osteoporosis?

Contrary to popular belief, you do not need dairy products to get sufficient calcium. Every natural food contains calcium. When you eat a healthy diet, rich in natural foods such as vegetables, beans, nuts, and seeds, it is impossible not to obtain sufficient calcium. In fact, the addition of more natural plant foods to the diet has been shown to have a powerful effect on increasing bone density and bone health.[13] All unprocessed, natural foods are calcium-rich, and green vegetables have particularly high levels. In fact, one four-ounce serving of steamed collards or kale has about the same amount of calcium as one cup of milk (six ounces of milk contains 225 mg of calcium). Take a look at a few other natural foods and their calcium levels.

Broccoli, cooked, two cups . . . . 190 mg

Collard greens, one cup . . . . .357 mg

Calcium-fortified orange juice (8 oz) . . 300 mg

Garbanzo beans, one cup . . . . 150 mg

Kale, cooked, one cup . . . . 180 mg

Lettuce, four cups . . . . 160 mg

Soybeans, one cup . . . . 175 mg

Sweet potato, two cups . . . . .160 mg

Tahini (sesame seed paste) two tbsp. . . .305 mg

Turnip greens, cooked, one cup . . . . . . 249 mg

Of course, when our calories come mostly from oil, sugar, flour, and animal meat, instead of unrefined plant foods such as these, it can appear that, without dairy, the diet would be too low in calcium. But, medical studies confirm that drinking cow's milk does not lead to stronger bones. Studies demonstrated that individuals who drank one glass or less of milk per week were at no greater risk of breaking a hip or forearm than were those who drank two or more glasses per week.[14] Researchers also found that high total calcium intake and milk consumption did not protect against osteoporotic fractures.[15]

Bone health is much more than just calcium. Vegetables, beans, fruits, and nuts are rich sources of calcium, potassium, Vitamin K, magnesium, and vegetable protein, as well as the phytochemicals and micronutrients that are gaining recognition as being important for bones. Calcium is an important component, but like protein, we don't need as much of it as most people think. The current U.S. daily calcium recommendation of 1200 to 1500 milligrams for postmenopausal women is an attempt to offset the ill-effects of the Standard American Diet which creates excessive calcium loss in the urine because it is so high in sodium and animal protein.

Even still, osteoporosis is occurring in epidemic proportions today. It affects 8 million American women and 2 million men, causing 1.5 million fractures each year. As many as 18 million additional Americans may have low bone density, which is a precursor to osteoporosis. Millions of women have been falsely led to believe that there is a correlation between osteoporosis and the inadequate intake of dairy foods. Women also must consider the extremely high concentration of saturated fat in milk and cheese (excluding skim-milk products). More than 50 percent of the calories in milk come from fat. Women are placing themselves at risk for heart disease and breast cancer by following the recommendations of the dairy industry.[16]

Osteoporosis is a disease caused by improper lifestyle and diet. To preserve bone density, many doctors and nutritionists recommend increased calcium intake, but, as I have described, this method fails to result in significant clinical improvements. The concept of a negative or positive nutrient balance must be understood before you can understand the physiologic mechanism underlying the development of osteoporosis. On a daily basis, the body absorbs calcium from the diet via the digestive tract and excretes calcium in the urine. A negative calcium balance means more calcium is excreted in the urine than is absorbed via digestion. A positive balance means more calcium is absorbed than is excreted. When you are in a negative balance, your body must obtain the needed calcium from the skeleton, the primary storehouse of this nutrient. Your body will not permit the level of calcium in your blood to drop below a certain, fixed amount. The continual depletion of bone calcium reserves over time results in progressive bone loss.

It is logical to think that a lower calcium intake could cause a negative calcium balance. However, studies on bone loss in different countries imply otherwise. Aging bone loss occurs in populations with widely varying calcium intakes. Countries whose populations have extremely high calcium intakes have the highest rates of osteoporosis in the world, and countries with low calcium intake often have low rates of osteoporosis. A positive calcium balance can occur with a lower calcium intake. What these studies show is that the primary culprit in osteo-porosis is not taking in too little calcium; it's when too much calcium is excreted through the urine.

Several dietary and lifestyle factors contribute to excessive urinary calcium loss and the resultant osteoporosis.

KEY FACTORS CAUSING OSTEOPOROSIS

A) **DIETS TOO HIGH IN ANIMAL PROTEIN AND LOW IN VEGETABLE PROTEIN** Meat and other high protein foods leave an acid residue in the blood that leads to bone dissolution. To neutralize this acid load, the body calls on its stores of calcium to provide basic calcium salts. Studies show that people with a high animal protein intake can develop a negative calcium balance, regardless of how much calcium is consumed. An important study demonstrated an increased bone loss and risk of hip fracture in those with a higher ratio of animal protein to vegetable protein. The researchers concluded that an increase in vegetable protein and a decrease in animal protein may decrease the risk of hip fractures in the elderly.[17] The recommendations are clear: green vegetables, beans, nuts, and seeds should be the major source of protein. It is important to note that later in life (after age 70), it is crucial to pay more attention to protein intake. At that point, both too much protein and too little protein are unfavorable to bone mass.[18]

B) **HIGH CONSUMPTION OF SALT AND/OR CAFFEINE** The consumption of large amounts of sodium and caffeine leads to unwanted excretion of calcium.[19] Exactly how this works is not completely understood, but both salt and caffeine increase the rate at which blood is filtered through the kidney. The increased filtering pressure and flow compromise the kidney's ability to return calcium supplies to the bloodstream.

C) SMOKING Nicotine can interfere with hormonal messages to the kidneys, inhibiting calcium reabsorption. The combination of smoking and drinking coffee or soft drinks, together with the dietary factors mentioned, makes the prevalence of osteoporosis in this country quite understandable. Dietary, health, and lifestyle components are working together to cause this drain of calcium.

D) VITAMIN D DEFICIENCY Recent research studies have corroborated the fact that most Americans are Vitamin D deficient. This deficiency occurred even among a majority of study subjects who were already taking a multivitamin with the standard 400 IUs of Vitamin D. More and more health authorities are recommending that an additional 400 to 800 IUs of Vitamin D be taken over and above the 400 typically present in a multiple vitamin.

E) VITAMIN A SUPPLEMENTS In high doses, Vitamin A (retinol) is associated with birth defects, and recent research suggests the dose that causes risk is much lower than previously thought. If Vitamin A is toxic to a person who is pregnant and potentially harmful to the developing baby, it can't be good for us the rest of the time. Research has shown it is linked to calcium loss in the urine and osteoporosis. For example, an important study found that subjects with a Vitamin A intake in the range of 1.5 mg had double the hip fracture rate of those with an intake in the range of .5 mg. For every 1 mg increase in Vitamin A consumption, hip fracture rates increased by 68 percent.[20] Most multivitamins contain about 5000 IUs of Vitamin A, which is equal to 1.5 mg. This means if you conform to the current recommendations, which have become outdated, and get your Vitamin A from supplements, you could be weakening your bones. Instead, the body can naturally self-fabricate Vitamin A by consuming beta-carotene and other carotenoids in real food. Vegetables such as carrots contain beta carotene, not Vitamin A, and the beta-carotene from vegetables does not lead to excessive Vitamin A formation or cause calcium loss.

F) **POOR PHYSICAL FITNESS** Our bones are continually dissolving old bone tissue and rebuilding new bone. Interestingly, our bone strength is directly proportional to our muscle strength. Bones, like muscles, respond to stress by becoming bigger and stronger, and, like muscles, bones weaken and literally shrink if not used. It is essential to exercise, and, in particular, to exercise the back. Studies have found that a back-strengthening exercise program can provide significant, long-lasting protection against spinal fractures in women at risk for osteoporosis.[21]

As you can see, increasing calcium intake will not prevent osteoporosis, and that is why so many Americans still suffer from it. While calcium is necessary in the diet, it is one of our greatest food myths that calcium has to be obtained from milk or other dairy products.

---

6. So, are milk and other dairy products a health hazard?

Few foods elicit such strong opinions as milk and dairy products. The dairy folks want you to believe that dairy is essential and that your bones will crumble if you don't drink milk. The anti-milk people talk about all the hormones and antibiotic residue in milk and consider it the most disease-promoting of all foods. There are exaggerations and distortions of the available research on both sides.

We can't look at all the pros and cons of dairy here, but there are some obvious conclusions. The typical American diet that is filled with processed foods and animal products is noticeably deficient in calcium and Vitamin D unless dairy is consumed or supplemented. However, dairy is not the only source of calcium, and, once you are eating a significant amount of calcium-rich plant matter, dairy products lose their status as the main source of calcium.

As you know from the evidence in this book, all animal products, including dairy, should be curtailed significantly, and those calories should be replaced with high-micronutrient, unprocessed plant foods.

When more vegetables are consumed, you get extra calcium and a cornucopia of phytochemicals that are not found in dairy. A secondary issue is that high saturated fat intake promotes heart disease and cancer. Dairy products, such as whole-milk, butter, and cheese are the foods that contribute the most saturated fat to the American diet. Any person seeking excellent health should restrict these foods in his or her diet. Skim-milk and other non-fat dairy products can be used as part of the small amount of allowable animal products consumed weekly. They are not foods that should be consumed liberally, and they should not be seen as health foods because they are not high in micronutrients and phytochemicals.

In addition to the other problems, there is evidence that the daily use of dairy can increase the risk of prostate cancer. Prostate cancer is now the single most common cancer among men in the United States. With the spread of our meat- and dairy-centered diet, it is on the rise in almost every country in the world. A meta-analysis of the best independent studies indicated that milk drinking men seem to have a 70 percent greater chance of developing cancer of the prostate.[22] This evidence exists in spite of the multiple studies that show that Vitamin D deficiency also increases the risk of prostate cancer. Since milk is fortified with Vitamin D, using it must have a significant negative effect that overwhelms the benefits from the added vitamin.

Overall, milk is not health food. If you enjoy some skim-milk or non-fat yogurt, I recommend you limit it, just as you would limit other animal products. If your diet is healthful, consuming little or no dairy won't be a problem, as long as you make sure you get adequate Vitamin D from other sources.

---

7. **I've read that the Mediterranean diet is the healthiest way to eat. Is that true?**

The Mediterranean diet describes a cuisine common to countries bordering the Mediterranean Sea. It is characterized by regular consumption of fruits, vegetables, cereals, legumes, and nuts. Red meat is rarely consumed, chicken and fish appear in small amounts, some yogurt and cheese is used, and red wine is very common. One of the most defining elements is the use of pasta and olive oil. Where most of the fat in the American diet comes from cheese, butter, meat, and dangerous trans fats, the principal fat source there is olive oil.

Compared to the American population, those eating this way in the Mediterranean region exhibit a lower risk of heart disease and common cancers. Heart attack rates are 25 percent lower, and the rate of obesity is about half of America's. The climate and fertile soil allow for many high-nutrient plants to grow, which makes most of the dishes rich in phytochemicals. That, in turn, accounts for the diet's protective effects. Nuts, particularly walnuts, are commonly used in the diet and they are a good source of omega-3 fats and other heart protective nutrients. The use of fish instead of meat also decreases saturated fat consumption and increases these beneficial fats. For these reasons, it is understandable why the Mediterranean diet is considered healthier than the SAD, but it is not without drawbacks. Studying its beneficial health outcomes—along with those of diets in other areas of the world such as Japan, rural China, Fiji, and Tibet— allows us to use the Mediterranean diet's culinary principals to make a diet deliciously varied and even more disease protective, while avoiding its problems.

One of the diet's main weak points is the use of pasta. The pasta intake should not be mimicked. There is very little difference between white bread and white pasta, and refined, white flour consumption has been linked to diabetes, obesity, heart disease, and various cancers. Whole grains are immensely superior to refined white flour, but they still should not be consumed as a major source of calories. The benefit of the Mediterranean style of eating is the large consumption of fruits and vegetables, not pasta.

The heavy use of olive oil is also problematic because all oil has 120 calories per tablespoon, and those calories can add up fast. It is better to use olive oil than butter or margarine, but olive oil can easily sabotage your success. Ounce for ounce, it is one of the most fattening, calorie-dense foods on the planet. Vegetables prepared in olive oil soak up more oil than you would think, which transforms them into high-calorie dishes. Heavy oil use will add fat to our waistlines, heightening the risk of disease and making losing weight more difficult.

To continue to consume foods prepared in oil and maintain a healthful, slender figure, dieters must carefully count calories from oil and eat small portions of it. Remember, oil does not contain the nutrients, fiber, and phytochemicals that were in the original seed or fruit. Compared to the calories it supplies, it contains few nutrients except a little Vitamin E and a negligible amount of phytochemicals. Olive oil is not a health food.

The Mediterranean people of past years ate lots of olive oil, but they also worked hard in the fields, walking about nine miles a day, often guiding a heavy plow. Today, people in the Mediterranean countries are over-weight, just like us. They still eat lots of olive oil, but their consumption of fruits, vegetables, and beans is down. Meat and cheese consumption has risen, and the physical activity level has plummeted. That way of living is not worth mimicking. The fast food and food technology indus tries have permeated most of the modern world. These people now follow a diet much like our own, and the rates of heart disease and obesity are skyrocketing in these countries. Living the *Eat For Health* way means that you use the valuable aspects of the Mediterranean diet, but leave behind its weaknesses, so that we do not merely reduce heart disease and obesity a little bit, but eliminate it all together. I want my risk and everyone else's reduced by almost 100 percent, which is possible when following the eating-style described within these pages.

8. Is it important to eat organically grown foods for good health?

The concern implicit in this question is about pesticides, and it is a real one. The Environmental Protection Agency has reported that the majority of pesticides now in use are probable or possible causes of cancer. Studies of farm workers who work with pesticides suggest a link between pesticide use and brain cancer, Parkinson's disease, multiple myeloma, leukemia, lymphoma, and cancers of the stomach and prostate.[23] However, does the low level of pesticides remaining on our food present much of a risk?

Some scientists argue that the extremely low level of pesticide residue remaining on produce is insignificant and that there are naturally occurring toxins in all natural foods that are more significant. The large amount of studies performed on the typical pesticide-treated produce have demonstrated that consumption of produce, whether organic or not, is related to lower rates of cancer and increased disease protection. In short, it is better to eat fruits and vegetables grown and harvested using pesticides than not to eat them at all. The health benefits of eating phytochemically-rich produce greatly outweigh any risks pesticide residues might pose. That said, it should be recognized that fruits and vegetables are not all subject to the same pesticide exposure. The below chart shows the pesticide breakdown by food, but it is alphabetized and not in order of pesticide content. Spinach, strawberries and celery have the most pesticide residue and are the most important foods to consume organically grown.

TWELVE FOODS WITH THE **MOST** PESTICIDES	TWELVE FOODS WITH THE **LEAST** PESTICIDES
1 Apples	1 Asparagus
2 Bell Peppers	2 Avocados
3 Celery	3 Bananas
4 Cherries	4 Broccoli
5 Imported Grapes	5 Cauliflower
6 Nectarines	6 Corn
7 Peaches	7 Kiwis
8 Pears	8 Mangos
9 Potatoes	9 Onions
10 Red Raspberries	10 Papaya
11 Spinach	11 Pineapple
12 Strawberries	12 Peas

If it is available, organic food is certainly your best bet to limit exposure to toxic chemicals. If you can eat only organic versions of the top 12 most contaminated fruits and vegetables, you can reduce your pesticide exposure by about 90 percent. In addition, organic foods usually have more nutrients than their conventional counterparts.[24] They also taste better and are generally better for farmers and the environment.

9. What nutritional supplements would be appropriate for a person eating healthfully?

One important principle you have learned is that when you eat nutrient-rich foods, you receive a symphony of phytochemicals. Supplements simply can't duplicate these. Even though adding powders, teas, and plant extracts may be beneficial for a person eating the deficient, conventional diet, they likely will not add a significant benefit to your excellent diet. Supplements should be supplements to a good diet; they should not be counted on instead of that diet. However, there are a few supplements that I do recommend, primarily DHA and a multivitamin with B12 and extra Vitamin D.

DHA is an omega-3 fatty acid found in fish, but because fish is so highly polluted in the modern world, I can't recommend eating enough to assure DHA adequacy. It is best to get most of your healthy fat intake from foods such as raw nuts and seeds. Ground flax seeds and walnuts are excellent sources of omega-3 fatty acids, but it is good nutritional assurance also to supplement your diet with DHA. It is also wise to add a DHA fat supplement to our diets, because many people require more DHA for optimal health and to delay age-related mental decline.

For years, I have found most fish oil and vegan DHA supplements to be foul-smelling and bad-tasting. I have even paid to have them tested for rancidity and the results were extremely high. Rancid fat can't be healthy, so I worked to make available a fresh, refrigerated DHA supplement— made from algae, not fish—which is appropriately named DHA Purity. Highly purified and freshly manufactured fish oil is an option as well.

Studies show you only need a very small amount to achieve healthy tissue levels of the long-chain, omega-3 fats, with even 100 mg a day of DHA being beneficial.[25]

Ensuring Vitamin B12 adequacy through a supplement is very important for all people, especially those restricting animal products. Vitamin D is also crucial if you do not live in a warm climate and get sufficient sunlight, so I recommend a multivitamin that contains Vitamins D and B12, as well as other nutrients such as iodine, zinc, and selenium. Many individuals, especially those not getting regular sun exposure, will require more Vitamin D than the 400 IUs present in a typical multivitamin. Vitamin D deficiency is the most common blood abnormality observed in my medical practice, but it is easily fixed by an additional Vitamin D supplement containing 800 IUs of the vitamin.

The main problem with taking many high dose multivitamins or other supplements is the high doses of Vitamin A, beta-carotene, iron, copper, Vitamin E, and Vitamin B6 that they contain. When supplemented, these items can have potentially negative effects on your health. Studies have shown these supplements are not beneficial and carry the following risks:

VITAMIN A—linked to calcium loss and osteoporosis[26]

BETA-CAROTENE—linked to higher rates of cancer in smokers[27]

VITAMIN B6—too much can be neurotoxic[28]

VITAMIN E—increased mortality[29]

IRON—higher rates of heart disease[30]

COPPER—higher rates of cancer and dementia[31]

Given these concerns, look for a multivitamin entirely free of Vitamin A and containing only small amounts of copper, iron, beta-carotene, and Vitamins E and B6. Supplemental guidelines and product recommendations can be found at **www.EatRightAmerica.com**.

10. Can I eat salmon? What about wild salmon?

As discussed in Chapter Thirteen, all fish contain high levels of pollutants–even salmon. But, recent studies showed dangerous chemicals were
ten-times higher in farm-raised salmon as compared to wild salmon. If
you're going to eat salmon, wild salmon is a better choice. Since there are
growing concerns about the high pollution and artificial colors used in
farm-raised salmon, wild salmon has become more desirable and its
prices have gone up. However, a 2005 article in the New York Times
reported that most fish labeled as wild Pacific or Alaskan salmon is just
farm-raised salmon with a lying label. The New York Times tested
salmon that was labeled as wild and sold in eight New York City stores
and found that most of the fish was farm-raised, not wild.[32]

They were able to tell the farm-raised from the wild salmon because of
the presence of an artificial, pink food dye manufactured by the pharmaceutical company Hoffman-La Roche. The company distributes their
trademarked SalmoFan, which is similar to paint store swatches, so fish
farmers can choose among various shades to make salmon have a pink-
orange color. Salmon in the wild have that color naturally from eating
pink crustaceans, but the commercially raised fish have a grey flesh from
eating fishmeal. Europeans are suspicious of the dye, which was linked
to retinal damage in people when taken as a sunless tanning pill.

Numerous studies also have found surprisingly high levels of PCBs and
dioxin in farm-raised salmon. American health officials' response was
that this level of contamination should not stop consumers from eating
salmon, but why should you unnecessarily expose yourself to known
toxic carcinogens? If you eat salmon, eat only the wild Alaskan variety.
If you eat fish once a week, use mostly the lower fat, less contaminated
fish, such as tilapia, flounder, scallops, trout, or sole, but I urge you to
eat fish infrequently since eating too much can promote heart disease,
cancer, and atrial fibrillation, as discussed previously.

11. What about alcohol? Should I be drinking red wine for my heart health?

Alcohol is not actually heart-healthy; it simply has anti-clotting effects, much like aspirin. Researchers have found that even moderate consumption of alcohol, including wine, interferes with blood clotting and thereby reduces heart attacks in high-risk populations, such as people who eat the typical, disease-promoting, American diet. Thinning the blood with alcohol or aspirin is not health-enhancing unless you are eating the typical heart-attack inducing diet. Once you are protected from heart attacks and strokes with nutritional excellence, the blood thinning only adds more risk in the form of gastrointestinal bleeding or a hemorrhagic stroke. Red wine contains some beneficial compounds such as flavonoids and resveratrol, a potent antioxidant in the skin of grapes associated with a number of health benefits. Of course, grapes, raisins, berries, and other plant foods also contain these beneficial compounds. One does not have to drink wine to gain these benefits.

Moderate drinking is defined as a maximum of one drink per day for women and two drinks for men. Consuming more than this is associated with increased fat around the waist and other significant health problems.[33] Even a moderate amount of alcohol may also increase the risk of breast cancer in susceptible women.[34] The other problem with alcohol, especially more than one drink a day, is it can create mild withdrawal sensations the next day. These sensations are commonly mistaken for hunger, which leads people to eat more than is necessary. Because of this, moderate drinkers are usually overweight. Furthermore, recent studies have also shown that even moderate alcohol consumption is linked to a significantly increased incidence of atrial fibrillation, a condition that can lead to stroke.[35]

Overall, it is safer to eat a diet that will not permit heart disease. Don't rely on alcohol to decrease the potential of blood to clot. Strive to avoid the detrimental effects of alcohol and protect yourself from heart disease with nutritional excellence. Having one alcoholic drink or one glass of wine is not a major risk, nor is it a major health asset. However, if consumed in excess, it can develop into a major health issue.

12. Will I experience any negative physical changes on this diet and if so how long will they last?

As your body's detoxification activities increase in the first week or two of this program, the symptoms of toxic hunger could increase. These feelings could include lightheadedness, fatigue, headaches, increased urination, sore throat, flatulence, and, very rarely, fever, body itching, and rashes. These uncomfortable sensations rarely last longer then one week and, even if they do, they will lessen with time.

Occasionally, people find it takes time for their digestive tract to adjust to all the additional raw fiber, and they experience an increase in gas or bloating or have looser stools. This is usually caused by the increased volume of raw vegetables and because you swallow more air when eating salads. It is remedied by chewing better so the air is out of the mouth before swallowing. Better chewing also breaks down the cells, making them easier to digest. For those with this problem, the amount of raw salad can be increased in a more gradual fashion. You can also eat less raw foods and more cooked vegetables, such as steamed zucchini, squash, brown rice, potato, and sweet potato. When the symptoms subside, gradually increase the amount of raw greens and cruciferous vegetables in your diet. Dried fruits, roasted nuts, and beans can also contribute to digestive problems at the beginning of transitioning to this way of eating. To combat these issues, use raw nuts, avoid dried fruit and other sweet substances, and soak beans in water overnight or eat them in smaller amounts until you adjust.

So, if you are troubled by digestive problems, try the following:

• Chew food better, especially salads.

- Eat beans in smaller amounts.

- Soak beans and legumes overnight before cooking.

- Avoid carbonated beverages.

- Do not overeat.

- Eat less raw vegetables and increase the raw vegetables gradually.

Be patient and give your body a little time to adjust to a different eating-style. Remember, your digestive tract can make the adjustments if allowed to do it gradually.

CHAPTER FIFTEEN

THE LAST WORD

Many eating-styles have been popularized in this country, and many of them have been investigated and have been shown to be more effective than the standard dietary advice of the American Heart Association for weight loss and lowering cholesterol. However, these diets have their pros and cons and are still not ideal. Most of them are designed to sell books and be popular, so they attempt to appeal to the existing American tastes and food preferences.

Commercial, social, and political interests govern the message imparted to Americans. Because of this, the solution to the American health problem is not going to come from the drug companies, the food industry, the medical industry, or governmental authorities. However, because of the explosion in sick and suffering individuals, and the dramatic increase in corporate health care costs, a fresh look at this problem with a different emphasis is a necessity. A revolution in health care as a result of corporate interest in improving employee health and performance and lowering costs may make it possible to have a dramatic improvement on our nation's health.

There are millions of individuals suffering with medical problems that could have been solved with nutritional excellence. They may have tried one after another of these popular diets and failed to lose weight. They may have given up, resigned to being in poor health. Worse, no one in authority told them that it was not that difficult to take back control of their health, reverse their medical conditions, remove the risk of heart disease and stroke, get off drugs, and get healthy again. They have been brainwashed by society and supported by their health professionals to think that drugs are the only approach to health care.

This program, which ranks the hierarchy of all foods based on their nutrient-per-calorie density and takes into account food addiction and toxic hunger, is different. The design is not founded on what will sell the most books, sound the most trendy, or win a popularity contest. Instead, it is designed to be the most effective at preventing and reversing disease and giving you amazing health for many, many years. Mathematically, it offers you the most disease-fighting nutrients in the lowest calorie load. In practice, it is an extremely powerful, therapeutic intervention that enables people to recover and maintain their health without prescription drugs.

As you know by now, the recommendations of *Eat For Health* are different from other eating-styles. High protein diets marketed for weight loss are meat or chicken-based. The USDA recommended diet is grain-based, as are most popular vegetarian diets. My eating-style has vegetables, beans, fruits, and nuts as its base, with an emphasis on a high volume of green vegetables. This eating-style has powerful disease reversal properties, is satisfying, and dramatically lowers body weight. It is designed around eating more healthy foods, not eating less food or counting calories. In practice, however, eating such large amounts of low-calorie, high-nutrient foods eventually results in people being satisfied with fewer calories. A recent study demonstrated that the average overweight person following this approach for two years lost 53 pounds and kept it off. This dietary approach to prevent and reverse chronic diseases is available for those who want the best health outcome. Many consider it the gold standard.

In my medical practice, patients following these nutritional recommendations routinely are able to cut their diabetic medications in half during the first month and get off them completely within six months. In a few months, most can gradually discontinue their blood pressure medications. Patients who have angina or known heart disease see dramatic improvement in their conditions. Within the first year on this program, it is typical for an at-risk patient's LDL cholesterol to drop over 100 points without drugs. I have had numerous patients who were scheduled for cardiac interventions, such as bypass surgeries or angioplasties, make complete recoveries from their conditions so that they no longer required these procedures.

A researcher from the National Institute of Health visited my office after reading and hearing about so many success stories of patients who have reversed their medical conditions. Dr. Tonja Nansel had the opportunity to see many new patients just starting out on this program, most of whom were able to dramatically reduce their medications within a few months. She also observed and took notes on patients who have been following my advice for years. John Pawlikoski was one such patient who had a typical story to tell:

> *I had a cardiac catheterization and my cardiologist told me I needed angioplasty. I went to Dr. Fuhrman instead, and, within two months, my chest pains were gone, my blood pressure returned to normal, and my cholesterol dropped 70 points! I went back to the cardiologist and he said, "Just keep listening to Dr. Fuhrman. You're doing great! You no longer need surgery."*

The interesting thing about John was that his first visit to me was 13 years ago. Dr. Nansel was impressed that John not only got rid of the blocked artery that caused his original chest pain without any medical interventions or surgery, he also lost 60 pounds and kept that weight off for all these years.

At the beginning, John required three medications to normalize his blood pressure. Today, at the age of 84, he is on no blood pressure or any other medication. His blood pressure gradually came down to 100/75 during the first two years on this program, and has remained there ever since. His LDL cholesterol began at 150, came down to 90, and stayed below that all these years. John maintains his great health and leads an extremely active life without any medication, which is unheard of for a man in his 80s in today's society. John Pawlikowski is not an isolated case. You too can get unbelievable results from this program. Don't ever forget that you have the freedom to choose what to eat and not to eat, and the freedom to have control over your health destiny. The choice is yours to live fully, live well, and live healthfully for the rest of your life.

I want you to succeed in following this program. It is easy to fall into a rut of ignoring our health. The momentary satisfaction of eating poor-quality food doesn't last very long, but the health-destructive ramifications of those decisions can permanently damage your body. If you find yourself in a pattern of self-defeating lifestyle choices and eating habits, you must examine why. It is important to examine our values, thoughts, feelings, and beliefs in order to replace food as the solution to our problems. You have made the choice to study this program. Now, make the choice to make it the way you live your life. Choose to be healthy and not depend on the rest of the world to say, "You're right." Don't depend on your doctor to assure you that you are in good health. It is likely he or she is plagued by the same addictions, nutritional misinformation, and societal pressures as you were. You must take charge, not ask for others' approval, and feel empowered that you can live and be healthy. There are some things you can't change, but now you know you can have dramatic control of your health destiny. This is a lifetime commitment. It can offer you a more pleasurable and better-quality life. You can feel good about every single step you have taken toward better health—even the small ones. Feel proud of your choices, maintain a positive attitude, and cultivate a positive, healthy influence on others.

I wish you a great life and enduring good health. It can be yours.

NOTES

INTRODUCTION

1 Fuhrman J, Sarter B, Campbell TC. Effect of a high-nutrient diet on long-term weight loss: a retrospective chart review. Altern Ther Health Med 2008;14(3):publication pending.

2 Svendsen M, Blomhoff R,Holme I, Tonstad S. The effect of an increased intake of vegetables and fruit on weight loss, blood pressure and antioxidant defense in subjects with sleep related breathing disorders. Euro J Cl in Nutr. 2007;61:1301–1311. Ello-Martin JA, Roe LS, Ledikwe JH, et al. Dietary energy density in the treatment of obesity: a year-long trial comparing 2 weight-loss diets. Am J Clin Nutr. 2007; 85(6):1465-1477. Howard BV, Manson JE, Stefanick ML, et al. Low-fat dietary pattern and weight change over 7 years: the Women's Health Initiative Dietary Modification Trial. JAMA. 2006; 295(1):39-49.

CHAPTER ONE

1 Bunyard LB, Dennis KE, Nicklas BJ. Dietary intake and changes in lipoprotein lipids in obese, postmenopausal women placed on an American Heart Association Step 1 diet. J Am Diet Assoc 2002 Jan;102(1):52-57.

2 Sharman MJ, Kraemer WJ, Love DM, et al. A ketogenic diet favorably affects serum biomarkers for cardiovascular disease in normal-weight men. J Nutr 2002 Jul;132(7):1879-1885.

3 Barnard ND, Scialli AR, Bertron P, et al. Effectiveness of a low-fat vegetarian diet in altering serum lipids in healthy premenopausal women. Am J Cardiol 2000 Apr 15;85(8):969-972.

4 Bemelmans WJ, Broer J, de Vries JH, et al. Impact of Mediterranean diet education versus posted leaflet on dietary habits and serum cholesterol in a high risk population for cardiovascular disease. Public Health Nutr. 2000 Sep;3(3):273-283.

5 Frolkis JP, Pearce GL, Nambi V, et al. Statins do not meet expectations for lowering low-density lipoprotein cholesterol levels when used in clinical practice. Am J Med 2002 Dec 1;113(8):625-629.

6 Jenkins DJ, Kendall CW, Popovich DG, et al. Effect of a very-high-fiber vegetable, fruit and nut diet on serum lipids and colonic function. Metabolism 2001 Apr;50(4):494-503.

7 Ward S, Lloyd JM, Pandor A, et al. A systematic review and economic evaluation of statins for the prevention of coronary events. Health Technol Assess. 2007;11(14):1-178.

8 Gardner CD, Coulston A, Chatterjee L, et al. The effect of a plant-based diet on plasma lipids in hypercholesterolemic adults: a randomized trial. Ann Intern Med. 2005;142(9):725-733.

9 Tucker KL, Hallfrisch J, Qiao N, et al. The combination of high fruit and vegetable and low saturated fat intakes is more protective against mortality in aging men than is either alone: the Baltimore Longitudinal Study of Aging. J Nutr. 2005;135(3):556-561.

10 Hu FB. Plant-based foods and prevention of cardiovascular disease: an overview. Am J Clin Nutr. 2003;78(3 Suppl):544S-551S.

11 Schauer PR, Burguera B, Ikramuddin S, et al. Effect of laparoscopic Roux-en Y gastric bypass on type 2 diabetes mellitus. Ann Surg. 2003;238(4):467-484; discussion 84-85.

12 Harder H, Dinesen B, Astrup A. The effect of a rapid weight loss on lipid profile and glycemic control in obese type 2 diabetic patients. Int J Obes Relat Metab Disord. 2004;28(1):180-182.

13 Barnard ND, Cohen J, Jenkins DJ, et al. A low-fat vegan diet improves glycemic control and cardiovascular risk factors in a randomized clinical trial in individuals with type 2 diabetes. Diabetes Care. 2006;29(8):1777-1783. Ford ES, Mokdad AH. Fruit and vegetable consumption and diabetes mellitus incidence among U.S. adults. Prev Med 2001;32(1):33-39.

Montonen J, Knekt P, Harkanen T, et al. Dietary patterns and the incidence of Type 2 Diabetes. Am J Epidem 2004;161(3):219-227.

14 Fuhrman J, Sarter B, Calabro DJ. Brief case reports of medically supervised, water-only fasting associated with remission of autoimmune disease. Altern-Ther-Health-Med. 2002 Jul-Aug; 8(4):110-112.

15 Nenonen M, Törrönen R, Häkkinen AS, et al. Antioxidants in vegan diet and rheumatic disorders. Toxicology. 2000;155(1-3):45-53. Müller H, de Toledo FW, Resch KL, et al. Fasting followed by vegetarian diet in patients with rheumatoid arthritis: a systematic review. Scand J Rheumatol. 2001;30(1):1-10. McDougall J, Bruce B, Spiller G, ct al. Effects of a very low-fat, vegan diet in subjects with rheumatoid arthritis. J Altern Complement Med. 2002;8(1):71-75. Darlington LG, Ramsey NW, Mansfield JR. Placebo-controlled, blind study of dietary manipulation therapy in rheumatoid arthritis. Lancet 1986;1(8475):236-238.

CHAPTER THREE

1 Lin RH. Potential synergy of phytochemicals in cancer prevention: mechanism of action. J Nutr. 2004;134(12 Suppl):3479S-3485S. Weiss JF, Landauer MR. Protection against ionizing radiation by antioxidant nutrients and phytochemicals. Toxicology 2003;189(1-2):1-20. Carratù B, Sanzini E. Biologically-active phytochemicals in vegetable food. Ann Ist Super Sanita. 2005; 41(1):7-16.

2 Hu FB. Plant-based foods and prevention of cardiovascular disease: an overview. Am J Clin Nutr. 2003 Sep;78(3 Suppl):544S-551S. Campbell TC, Parpia B, Chen J. Diet, lifestyle, and the etiology of coronary artery disease: the Cornell China study. Am J Cardiol 1998 Nov 26;82(10B):18T-21T. Fujimoto N, Matsubayashi K, Miyahara T, et al. The risk factors for ischemic heart disease in Tibetan highlanders. Jpn Heart J. 1989 Jan;30(1):27-34. Tatsukawa M, Sawayama Y, Maeda N, et al. Carotid atherosclerosis and cardiovascular risk factors: a comparison of residents of a rural area of Okinawa with residents of a typical suburban area of Fukuoka, Japan. Atherosclerosis 2004;172(2):337-343.

3 Hu FB, Willett WC. Optimal diets for prevention of coronary heart disease. JAMA 2002 Nov 27;288(20):2569-2578. Esselstyn CB. Resolving the Coronary Artery Disease Epidemic Through Plant-Based Nutrition. 2001 Autumn;4(4):171-177.

4 Oregon State University, The Linus Pauling Institute, Micronutrient Research for Optimum Health, Isothiocyanates, www.oregonstate.edu/infocenter/phytochemicals/isothio

5 Xianli W, Beecher G, Holden J, et al. Lipophilic and Hydrophilic Antioxidant Capacities of Common Foods in the United States. Journal of Agricultural and Food Chemistry 2004;52:4026-4037.

6 Dietary Reference Intakes for Vitamin C, Vitamin E, Selenium and Caroteinoids. The National Academies 2000. McBride J. Agricultural Research; Can Foods Forestall Aging?; February, 1999.

CHAPTER FOUR

1 Gardner CD, Coulston A, Chatterjee L, et al. The effect of a plant-based diet on plasma lipids in hypercholesterolemic adults: a randomized trial. Ann Intern Med. 2005;142(9):725-733. Tucker KL, Hallfrisch J, Qiao N, et al. The combination of high fruit and vegetable and low saturated fat intakes is more protective against mortality in aging men than is either alone: the Baltimore Longitudinal Study of Aging. J Nutr. 2005;135(3):556-561.

2 Vasan RS, Beiser A, Seshadri S, et al. Residual lifetime risk for developing hypertension in middle-aged women and men: The Framingham Heart Study. JAMA 2002;287(8):1003-1010.

3 Black HR. The burden of cardiovascular disease: following the link from hypertension to myocardial infarction and heart failure. Am J Hypertens. 2003;16(9 Pt 2):4S-6S.

4 Freis ED. Salt, volume and the prevention of hypertension. Circulation 1976;54:589.

5 Ziegler RG, Hoover RN, Pike MC, et al. Migration Patterns and Breast Cancer

Risk in Asian-American Women. J. Natl. Cancer Inst.1993;85:1819-1827.

CHAPTER SIX

1 Giles LC. Effect of social networks on 10 year survival in very old Australians: the Australian longitudinal study of aging. Journal of Epidemiology and Community Health July 2005;59(7):574-579.

2 Lea EJ, Crawford D, Worsley A. Consumers' readiness to eat a plant-based diet. European Journal of Clinical Nutrition 2006;60:342–351.

3 Mattson MP, Wan R. Beneficial effects of intermittent fasting and caloric restriction on the cardiovascular and cerebrovascular systems. J Nutr Biochem. 2005;16(3):129-137.

4 Bouchard C. The causes of obesity: advances in molecular biology but stagnation on the genetic front. Diabetologia 1996;39(12):1532-1533.

5 Weinsier RL, Krumdieck CL. Dairy foods and bone health: examination of the evidence. Am J Clin Nutr 2000;72:681–689.

6 Sinnett PF, Whyte HM. Epidemiological studies in total highland population, Tukisenta, New Guinea. Cardiovascular disease and relevant clinical, electrocardiography, radiological and biochemical findings. J Chron Diseases 1973;26:265. Campbell TC, Parpia B, Chen J. Diet, lifestyle and the etiology of coronary artery disease: The Cornell China Study. Am J Card 1998;82(10B):18T-21T. Miller K. Lipid values in Kalahari Bushman. Arch Intern Med 1968;121:414. Breslow JL. Cardiovascular disease myths and facts. Cleve Clin J Med. 1998;65(6):286-287.

7 Commenges D, Scotet V, Renaud S, et al. Intake of flavonoids and risk of dementia. Eur J Epidemiol. 2000;16(4):357-363. Otsuka M, Yamaguchi K, Ueki A. Similarities and differences between Alzheimer's disease and vascular dementia from the viewpoint of nutrition. Ann NY Acad Sci. 2002;977:155-161. Nash DT, Fillit H. Cardiovascular disease risk factors and cognitive impairment. Am J Cardiol. 2006;97(8):1262-1265.

8 Golay A, Guy-Grand B. Are diets fattening? Ann Endocrinol 2002;63(6):2.

CHAPTER SEVEN

1 Maguire EA, Spiers HJ, Good CD, et al. Navigation expertise and the human hippocampus: a structural brain imaging analysis. Hippocampus. 2003;13(2):250-259.

CHAPTER NINE

1 He FJ, MacGregor GA. Blood pressure is the most important cause of death and disability in the world. European Heart Journal Supplements 2007;9:B23-B28.

2 Seals DR, Tanaka H, Clevenger CM, et al Blood pressure reductions with exercise and sodium restriction in postmenopausal women with elevated systolic pressure: role of arterial stiffness. J Am Coll Cardiol, 2001; 38:506-513

3 Cook NR, Cutler JA, Obarzanek E, et al. Long term effects of dietary sodium reduction on cardiovascular disease outcomes: observational follow-up of the trials of hypertension prevention (TOHP). BMJ 2007; 334(7599):885.

4 Tuomilehto J, Jousilahti P, Rastenyte D, et al. Urinary sodium excretion and cardiovascular mortality in Finland: a prospective study. Lancet 2001;357:848-851.

5 Tirschwell DL, Smith NL, Heckbert SR, et al. Association of cholesterol with stroke risk varies in stroke subtypes and patient subgroups. Neurology 2004;63(10):1868-1875.

6 Duwe AK, Fitch M, Ostwald R, et al. Depressed Natural Killer and Lecithin-Induced Cell-Mediated Cytotoxicity in Cholesterol-Fed Guinea Pigs. J Nat Cancer Inst 1984;72(2):333-338.

7 Roberts JC, Moses C, Wilkins RH. Autopsy Studies in Atherosclerosis. I. Distribution and Severity of Atherosclerosis in Patients Dying without Morphologic Evidence of Atherosclerotic Catastrophe. Circulation 1959;20:511. Berenson GS, et al. Bogalusa Heart Study: A long-term community study of a rural biracial (black/white) population. Am J Med Sci 2001;322(5):267-274.

8 Huxley R, Lewington S, Clarke R. Cholesterol, coronary heart disease and stroke: a review of published evidence from observational studies and randomized controlled trials. Semin Vasc Med. 2002;2(3):315-323.

9 Hu FB, Manson JE, Willett WC. Types of dietary fat and risk of coronary heart disease: a critical review. J Am Coll Nutr. 2001;20(1):5-19.

10 Composition of Foods - Raw-Processed-Prepared, Agriculture Handbook 8. Series and Supplements. United States Department of Agriculture, Human Nutrition Information Service, Minnesota Nutrition Data System (NDS) software, developed by the Nutrition Coordinating Center, University of Minnesota, Minneapolis, MN. Food Database version 5A, Nutrient Database version 20, USDA Nutrient Database for Standard Reference. Release 14 at www.nal.usda.gov.fnic

11 Okuyama H, Kobayashi T, Watanabe S. Dietary fatty acids—the N-6/N-3 balance and chronic elderly diseases. Excess linoleic acid and relative N-3 deficiency syndrome seen in Japan. Prog Lipid Res. 1996 Dec;35(4):409-457.

12 Itabe H. Oxidized Phospholipids as a New Landmark in Atherosclerosis. Prog Lipid Research 1998;37(2/3):181-207.

13 Tucker KL, Hallfrisch J, Qiao N, et al. The combination of high fruit and vegetable and low saturated fat intakes is more protective against mortality in aging men than is either alone: the Baltimore Longitudinal Study of Aging. J Nutr. 2005;135(3):556-561.

14 Larsson SC, Rafter J, Holmberg L, et al. Red meat consumption and risk of cancers of the proximal colon, distal colon and rectum: the Swedish Mammography Cohort. Int J Cancer 2005; 113(5):829-834. Larsson SC, Håkanson N, Permert J, Wolk A. Meat, fish, poultry and egg consumption in relation to risk of pancreatic cancer: a prospective study. Int J Cancer 2006; 118(11):2866-2870.

15 Chao A, Thun JT, Connell CJ, et al. Meat Consumption and Risk of Colorectal Cancer JAMA 2005;293:172-182.

16 Sesink AL, Termont DS, Kleibeuker JH, Van der Meer R. Red meat and colon cancer: dietary haem-induced colonic cytotoxicity and epithelial hyperproliferation are inhibited by calcium. Carcinogenesis 2001;22(10):1653-1659. Hughes R, Cross AJ, Pollock JR, Bingham S. Dose-dependent effect of dietary meat on endogenous colonic N-nitrosation. Carcinogenesis 2001; 22(1):199-202.

17 Melita A, Jain AC, Mehta MC, Billie M. Caffeine and cardiac arrhythmias, An experimental study in dogs with review of literature. Acta Cardiol 1997;52(3):273-283. Nurminen MI, Niittymen L, Retterstol I, et al. Coffee, caffeine, and blood pressure: a critical review. Eur J Clin Nutr 1999;53(11):831-839. Christensen B, Mosdol A, Retterstol I, et al. Abstention from filtered coffee reduces the concentration of plasma homo-cysteine and serum cholesterol-a randomized controlled trial. Am J Clin Nutr 2001;74(3):302-307. Higdon JV, Frei B. Coffee and health: a review of recent human research.Crit Rev Food Sci Nutr. 2006; 46(2):101-123. Hallström H, Wolk A, Glynn A, Michaëlsson K. Coffee, tea and caffeine consumption in relation to osteoporotic fracture risk in a cohort of Swedish women.Osteoporos Int. 2006;17(7):1055-1064.

18 Spiegel K, Leproult R, Van Cauter EV. Impact of sleep debt on metabolic and endocrine function. Lancet 1999;354(9188);1435-1439.

19 Lucero J, Harlow BI, Berbieri RI, et al. Early follicular phase hormone levels in relation to patterns of alcohol, tobacco and coffee use. Fertile Steril 2001;76(4):723-729.

20 Colantuoni C, Rada P, McCarthy J, et al. Evidence that intermittent, excessive sugar intake causes endogenous opioid dependence. Obes Res. 2002;10(6):478-488. Rada P, Avena NM, Hoebel BG. Daily bingeing on sugar repeatedly releases dopamine in the accumbens shell. Neuroscience 2005;134(3):737-744.

CHAPTER TEN

1 Kahn HA, Phillips RI, Snowdon DA, Choi W. Association between reported diet and all cause mortality: Twenty-one year follow up on 27,530 adult Seventh-Day Adventists. Am J Epidemiol 1984;119:775-787.

2 Hu FB, Stampfer MJ. Nut consumption and risk of coronary heart disease: a review of epidemiologic evidence. Curr Atheroscler Rep 1999 Nov;1(3):204-209.

3 Ellsworth JL, Kushi LH, Folsom AR, et al. Frequent nut intake and risk of death from coronary heart disease and all causes in postmenopausal women: the Iowa Women's Health Study.

Nutr Metab Cardiovasc Dis. 2001;11(6):372-377. Kris-Etherton PM, Zhao G, Binkoski AE, et al. The effects of nuts on coronary heart disease risk. Nutr Rev. 2001;59(4):103-111.

4 Simopoulos AP. Essential fatty acids in health and chronic disease. Am J Clin Nutr. 1999;70 (3):56S-69S.

5 Rajaram S, Sabat AJ. Nuts, body weight and insulin resistance.Br J Nutr 2006;96 Suppl 2:S79-S86. Sabat AJ. Nut consumption and body weight. Am J Clin Nutr 2003;78(3 Suppl):647S-650S. Bes-Rastrollo M, Sabat AJ, Gamez-Gracia E, et al. Nut consumption and weight gain in a Mediterranean cohort: The SUN study. Obesity 2007;15(1):107-116. Garc-a-Lorda P, Megias Rangil I, Salas-Salvada J. Nut consumption, body weight and insulin resistance. Eur J Clin Nutr 2003;57 Suppl 1:S8-11. Meg-as-Rangil I, Garc-a-Lorda P, Torres-Moreno M, et al. Nutrient content and health effects of nuts. Arch Latinoam Nutr 2004;54(2 Suppl 1):83-86.

6 Lovejoy JC. The impact of nuts on diabetes and diabetes risk.Curr Diab Rep 2005; 5(5):379-84. Jiang R, Manson JE, Stampfer MJ, Liu S, Willett WC, Hu FB. Nut and peanut butter consumption and risk of type 2 diabetes in women. JAMA 2002; 288(20):2554-2560.

7 Tsai CJ, Leitzmann MF, Hu FB, Willett WC, Giovannucci EL. Frequent nut consumption and decreased risk of cholecystectomy in women. Am J Clin

Nutr 2004; 80(1):76-81. Tsai Cj, Leitzmann Me, Hu FB, et al. A prospective cohort study of nut consumption and the risk of gallstone disease in men. Am J Epid 2004;160(10):961-968.

CHAPTER THIRTEEN

1 Link LB, Potter JD. Raw versus cooked vegetables and cancer risk. Cancer Epidemiol Biomarkers Prev. 2004;13(9):1422-1435. Franceschi S, Parpinel M, La Vecchia C, et al. Role of different types of vegetables and fruit in the prevention of cancer of the colon, rectum, and breast. Epidemiology 1998;9(3):338-341. McEligot AJ, Rock CL, Shanks TG, et al. Comparison of serum carotenoid responses between women consuming vegetable juice and women consuming raw or cooked vegetables. Cancer Epidemiol Biomarkers Prev. 1999;8(3):227-231.

2 Key TJA, Thorogood M, Appleby PN, Burr ML. Dietary habits and mortality in 11,000 vegetarians and health conscious people: results of a 17-year follow up. BMJ 1996;313:775-779.

3 Rolls BJ, Roe LS, Meegns JS. Salad and satiety: energy density and portion size of a first-course salad affect energy intake at lunch. J Am Diet Assoc. 2004;104(10):1570-1576.

4 Unlu NZ, Bohn T, Clinton SK, Schwartz SJ. Carotenoid absorption from salad and salsa by humans is enhanced by the addition of avocado or avocado oil. J Nutr. 2005;135(3):431-436.

5 Steinmetz KA, Potter JD. Vegetables, fruit, and cancer prevention: a review. J Am Diet Assoc. 1996;96(10):1027-1039. Genkinger JM, Platz EA, Hoffman SC, et al. Fruit, vegetable, and antioxidant intake and all-cause, cancer, and cardiovascular disease mortality in a community-dwelling population in Washington County, Maryland. Am J Epidemiol. 2004;160(12):1223-1233.

6 Bugianesi R, Salucci M, Leonardi C, et al. Effect of domestic cooking on human bioavailability of naringenin, chlorogenic acid, lycopene and beta-carotene in cherry tomatoes. Eur J Nutr. 2004; 43(6):360-366.

7 Jansen MC, Bueno-de-Mesquita HB, Feskens EJ, et al. Quantity and variety of fruit and vegetable consumption and cancer risk. Nutr Cancer. 2004;48(2):142-148.

8 Lau FC, Shukitt-Hale B, Joseph JA. The beneficial effects of fruit polyphenols on brain aging. Neurobiol Aging. 2005;26(Suppl 1):128-132.

9 Gorinstein S, Caspi A, Libman I, et al. Red grapefruit positively influences serum triglyceride level in patients suffering from coronary atherosclerosis: studies in vitro and in humans. J Agric Food Chem. 2006;54(5):1887-1892. Aviram M, Rosenblat M, Gaitini D, et al. Pomegranate juice consumption for 3 years by patients with carotid artery stenosis reduces common carotid intima-media thickness, blood pressure and LDL oxidation. Clin Nutr. 2004;23(3):423-433. Duttaroy AK, Jørgensen A. Effects of kiwi fruit consumption on platelet aggregation and plasma lipids in healthy human volunteers. Platelets 2004;15(5):287-292.

10 Liu S, Sesso HD, Manson JE, et al. Is intake of breakfast cereals related to total and cause-specific mortality in men? Am J Clin Nutr. 2003;77(3):594-599. Liu S. Intake of refined carbohydrates and whole grain foods in relation to risk of type 2 diabetes mellitus and coronary heart disease. J Am Coll Nutr. 2002;21(4):298-306. Gross LS, Li L, Ford ES, Liu S. Increased consumption of refined carbohydrates and the epidemic of type 2 diabetes in the United States: an ecologic assessment. Am J Clin Nutr. 2004;79(5):774-779. Prentice AM. The emerging epidemic of obesity in developing countries. Int J Epidemiol. 2006;35(1):93-99.

11 Bravi F, Bosetti C, Dal Maso L, et al. Macronutrients, fatty acids, cholesterol, and risk of benign prostatic hyperplasia. Urology 2006;67(6):1205-1211.

12 Halton TL, Willett WC, Liu S, et al. Potato and french fry consumption and risk of type 2 diabetes in women. Am J Clin Nutr. 2006;83(2):284-290.

13 Hightower JM, Moore D. Mercury levels in high-end consumers of fish. Environmental Health Perspectives 2003;111(4):604-608.

14 Mahaffey KR, Clickner RP, Bodurow CC. Blood organic mercury and dietary mercury intake: National Health and Nutrition Examination Survey, 1999 and 2000. Env Health Persp 2004;112(5):562-570.

15 Diakovich MP, Efimova NV. Assessment of health risks upon exposure to mentholated mercury. Gig Sanit 2001;2:49-51.

16 Solonen JT, Seppanen K, Nyyssonen K, et al. Intake of mercury from fish, lipid peroxidation and the risk of myocardial infarction and coronary cardiovascular, and any death in Easter Finnish Men. Circulation 1995;91:645-655. Peitinen P, Ascherio A, Krohonen P, et al. Intake of fatty acids and risk of coronary heart disease in a cohort of Finnish men. Am J Epidemiol 1997;145:876-887.

17 Stripp C, Overvad K, Christensen J, et al. Fish intake is positively associated with breast cancer incidence rate. J Nutr 2003;133(11):3664-3669.

18 Glattre E, Haldorsen T, Berg JP, et al. Norwegian case-control study testing the hypothesis that seafood increase the risk of thyroid cancer. Cancer Causes and Control 1993;4:11-16.

CHAPTER FOURTEEN

1 Bouchard C. The causes of obesity: advances in molecular biology but stagnation on the genetic front. Diabetologia 1996;39(12):1532-1533.

2 Christakis NA, Fowler JH. The spread of obesity in a large social network over 32 years. NEJM 2007;327(4):370-379.

3 Sinnett PF, Whyte HM. Epidemiological studies in total highland population, Tukisenta, New Guinea. Cardiovascular disease and relevant clinical, electrocardiography, radiological and biochemical findings. J Chron Diseases 1973;26:265. Campbell TC, Parpia B, Chen J. Diet, lifestyle and the etiology of coronary artery disease: The Cornell China Study. Am J Card 1998;82(10B):18T-21T. Miller K. Lipid values in Kalahari Bushman. Arch Intern Med 1968;121:414. Breslow JL. Cardiovascular disease myths and facts. Cleve Clin J Med. 1998;65(6):286-287.

4 Palmieri L, Donfrancesco C, Giampaoli S, et al. Favorable cardiovascular risk profile and 10-year coronary heart disease incidence in women and men: results from the Progetto CUORE. Eur J Cardiovasc Prev Rehabil. 2006;13(4):562-570.

5 Commenges D, Scotet V, Renaud S, et al. Intake of flavonoids and risk of dementia. Eur J Epidemiol. 2000;16(4):357-363. Otsuka M, Yamaguchi K, Ueki A. Similarities and differences between Alzheimer's disease and vascular dementia from the viewpoint of nutrition. Ann N Y Acad Sci. 2002;977:155-161. Nash DT, Fillit H. Cardiovascular disease risk factors and cognitive impairment. Am J Cardiol. 2006;97(8):1262-1265.

6 Rraser GE, Shavlik DJ.Ten years of life: is it a matter of choice? Arch Intern Med 2001;161(13):1645-1652.

7 Singh PN, Sebate J, Fraser Ge. Does low meat consumption increase life expectancy in humans? Am J Clin Nutr 2003;78(3Suppl):526S-532S.

8 Campbell TC, Parpia B, Chen J. Diet, lifestyle, and the etiology of coronary artery disease: the Cornell China study. Am J Cardiol. 1998; 82(10B):18T-21T.

9 Robbins J. Healthy At 100. Random House, New York 2006

10 Rose W. The amino acid requirements of adult man. Nutritional Abstracts and Reviews 1957;27:631.

11 Hardage M. Nutritional studies of vegetarians. Journal of the American Dietetic Association 1966;48:25.

12 Baron S. NIOSII study refutes myth of early death. The New Audible (National Football League Player Association Newsletter) 1994;17(1):1-2.

13 New SA, Robins SP, Campbell MK, et al. Dietary influences on bone mass and bone metabolism: further evidence of a positive link between fruit and vegetable consumption and bone health? Am J Clin Nutr 2000;71(1):142-151.

14 Owusu W, Willett WC, Feskanich D, Ascherio A, Spiegelman D, Colditz GA. Calcium intake and the incidence of forearm and hip fractures among men.

J Nutr 997;127:1782-1787. Feskanich D, Willett WC, Stampfer MJ, Colditz GA. Milk, dietary calcium, and bone fractures in women: a 12-year prospective study. Am J Public Health 1997;87:992-997.

15 Feskanich D, Willett WC, Colditz GA. Calcium, vitamin D, milk consumption and hip fractures: a prospective study among post-menopausal women. Am J Clin Nutr 2003:77(2):504-511.

16 Boyd NF, Stone J, Vogt KN, et al. Dietary fat and breast cancer risk revisited: a meta-analysis of the published literature. Br J Cancer. 2003;89(9):1672-1685.

17 Sellmeyer DE, Stone KL, Sebastian A, Cummings SR. A high ratio of dietary animal to vegetable protein increases the rate of bone loss and the risk of fracture in postmenopausal women. Study of Osteoporotic Fractures Research Group. Am J Clin Nutr. 2001;73(1):118-122.

18 Devine A, Dick IM, Islam AF, Dhaliwal SS, Prince RL. Protein consumption is an important predictor of lower limb bone mass in elderly women. Am J Clin Nutr. 2005;81(6):1423-1428.

19 Teucher B, Fairweather-Tait S. Dietary sodium as a risk factor for osteoporosis: where is the evidence? Proc Nutr Soc. 2003;62(4):859-866. Rapuri PB, Gallagher JC, Kinyamu HK, Ryschon KL. Caffeine intake increases the rate of bone loss in elderly women and interacts with vitamin D receptor genotypes. Am J Clin Nutr. 2001;74(5):694-700. Hallström H, Wolk A, Glynn A, Michaëlsson K. Coffee, tea and caffeine consumption in relation to osteoporotic fracture risk in a cohort of Swedish women. Osteoporos Int. 2006;17(7):1055-1064.

20 Whiting SJ, Lemke B. Excess retinol intake may explain the high incidence of osteoporosis in northern Europe. Nutr Rev 1999;57(6):192-195. Melhus H, Michaelson K, Kindmark A, et al. Excessive dietary intake of vitamin A is associated with reduced bone mineral density and increased risk of hip fracture. Ann Intern Med. 1998;129(10):770-778.

21 Sinaki M, Itoi E, Wahner HW, et al. Stronger back muscles reduce the incidence of vertebral fractures: a prospective 10 year follow-up of post-menopausal women. Bone. 2002;30(6):836-841.

22 Qin LQ, Xu JY, Wang PY, et al. Milk consumption is a risk factor for prostate cancer: meta-analysis of case-control studies. Nutr Cancer. 2004;48(1):22-27.

23 Sanderson W.T., Talaska G, Zaebst D, et al. Pesticide prioritization for a brain cancer case-control study. Environ Res. 1997;74(2):133-144. Zahm SH, Blair A. Cancer among migrant and seasonal farmworkers: an epidemiologic review and research agenda. Am J Ind Med 1993;24(6): 753-766.

24 Worthington V. Nutritional quality of organic versus conventional fruits, vegetables and grains. J Alt Coml Med 2001;7(2):161-173. Grinder-Pederson L, Rasmussen SE, Bugel S, et al. Effect of diets based on foods from conventional versus organic production on intake and excretion of flavonoids and markers of antioxidative defense in humans. J Agric Food Chem. 2003;51(19): 5671-5676

25 Geppert J, Kraft V, Demmelmair H, Koltzko B. Docosahexaenoic acid supplementation in vegetarians effectively increases omega-3 index: a randomized trial. Lipids 2005;40(8):807-814.

26 Lim LS, Harnack LJ, Lazovich D, Folsom AR. Vitamin A intake and the risk of hip fracture in postmenopausal women: the Iowa Women's Health Study. Osteoporos Int. 2004;15(7):552-559. Crandall C. Vitamin A intake and osteoporosis: a clinical review. J Womens Health (Larchmt). 2004;13(8):939-953.

27 Virtamo J, Pietinen P, Huttunen JK, et al. Incidence of cancer and mortality following alpha-tocopherol and beta-carotene supplementation: a postintervention follow-up. JAMA. 2003;290(4):476-485. Touvier M, Kesse E, Clavel-Chapelon F, Boutron-Ruault MC. Dual Association of beta-carotene with risk of tobacco-related cancers in a cohort of French women. J Natl Cancer Inst. 2005;97(18):1338-1344. Black HS. Pro-carcinogenic activity of beta-carotene, a putative systemic photoprotectant. Photochem Photobiol Sci. 2004;3(8):753-758.

28 De Kruijk JR, Notermans NC. Sensory disturbances caused by multivitamin preparations. Ned Tijdschr Geneeskd. 2005;149(46):2541-2544.

29 Miller ER, Pastor-Barriuso R, Dalal D, et al. Meta-analysis: high-dosage vitamin E supplementation may increase all-cause mortality. Ann Intern Med. 2005;142(1):37-46.

30 De Valk B, Marx JJ. Iron, atherosclerosis, and ischemic heart disease. Arch Intern Med. 1999; 159(14):1542-1548.

31 Leone N, Courbon D, Ducimetiere P, Zureik M. Zinc, copper, and magnesium and risks for all-cause, cancer, and cardiovascular mortality. Epidemiology 2006;17(3):308-314. Senesse P, Meance S, Cottet V, et al. High dietary iron and copper and risk of colorectal cancer: a case-control study in Burgundy, France. Nutr Cancer. 2004;49(1):66-71. Dalla Nora E, Smorgon C, Mari E, Atti AR, et al. Trace elements and cognitive impairment: an elderly cohort study. Arch Gerontol Geriatr Suppl. 2004;(9):393-402.

32 Burros, M. Stores say wild salmon, but tests say farm bred. New York Times April 10, 2005. page 1.

33 Dallongeville J, Marecaux N, Ducmetiere P, et al. Influence of alcohol consumption and various beverages on waist girth and waist-to-hip ratio on a sample of French men and women. J Obes. Relat. Metab. Disord. 1998;22(12):1178-1183.

34 Dumitrescu RG, Shields PG. The etiology of alcohol-induced breast cancer. Alcohol. 2005; 35(3):213-225.

35 Frost L, Vestergaard P. Alcohol and risk of atrial fibrillation or flutter: a cohort study. Arch Intern Med. 2004;164(18):1993-1998. Mukamal KJ, Tolstrup JS, Friberg J, et al. Alcohol consumption and risk of atrial fibrillation in men and women: the Copenhagen City Heart Study. Circulation. 2005;112(12):1736-1742.

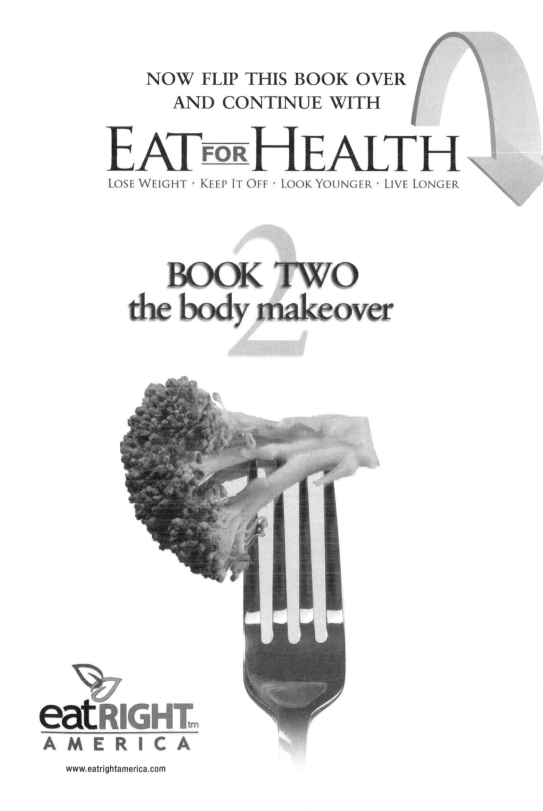

NOW FLIP THIS BOOK OVER
AND CONTINUE WITH

EAT FOR HEALTH

LOSE WEIGHT · KEEP IT OFF · LOOK YOUNGER · LIVE LONGER

BOOK TWO
the body makeover

eatRIGHT™
AMERICA

www.eatrightamerica.com

YUMMY BANANA-OAT BARS

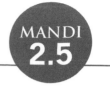

MANDI
2.5

Serves: 8 — Prep Time: 10 minutes

INGREDIENTS

2 cups quick old fashioned oats (not instant)

1/2 cup shredded coconut

1/2 cup raisins or chopped dates

1/4 cup chopped walnuts

2 large ripe bananas, mashed

1/4 cup unsweetened applesauce (optional)

1 tablespoon date sugar (optional)

> ADD THE APPLESAUCE AND DATE SUGAR FOR A SWEETER, MOISTER VERSION OF THESE BARS.

DIRECTIONS

Preheat oven to 350 degrees.

Mix ingredients together in a large bowl.

Press dough in a 9"X 9" baking pan and bake for 30 minutes.

Cool on wire rack. When cool, slice into squares or bars and serve.

One Serving Contains:
CALORIES 250; PROTEIN 7.7g; CARBOHYDRATE 41.9g; FAT 6.9g; SODIUM 3.3mg

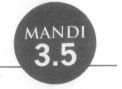

WILD APPLE CRUNCH

Serves: 8 — Prep Time: 15 minutes

INGREDIENTS

6 apples, peeled and sliced

3/4 cup chopped walnuts

8 dates, chopped

1 cup currants or raisins

3/4 cup water

1/2 teaspoon cinnamon

1/4 teaspoon nutmeg

juice of 1 orange

> YOU CAN ALSO SIMMER THIS IN A COVERED POT FOR 30 MINUTES ON TOP OF THE STOVE, STIRRING OCCASIONALLY.

DIRECTIONS

Preheat oven to 375 degrees.

Combine all ingredients except the orange juice. Place in a baking pan and drizzle the orange juice on top.

Cover and bake at 375 degrees for about one hour until all ingredients are soft, stirring occasionally.

One Serving Contains:
CALORIES 207.4; PROTEIN 4.7g; CARBOHYDRATE 37.3g; FAT 7.5g; SODIUM 4.2mg

"Remember ... the prescription is nutrition."

~ JOEL FUHRMAN, M.D.

For more recipes and support visit

www.EatRightAmerica.com